Communicating with Patients

PSYCHOLOGY AND MEDICINE SERIES

Series Editor: Donald Marcer, Department of Psychology, University of Southampton

Already Available:

Biofeedback and Related Therapies in Clinical Practice *Donald Marcer*
Psychological Problems in Primary Health Care *Eric Button*
Psychology and Diabetes: Psychosocial Factors in Management and
    Control *Richard W. Shillitoe*

In Preparation:

Family Systems in Health and Illness *Arlene Vetere*
Understanding Stress: A Psychological Perspective for the Health
    Professions *Cary L. Cooper and Val Sutherland*
Breaking Bad News? Giving Diagnoses to Patients *Ian Robinson*
Chronic Pain: Multidisciplinary Approaches to Treatment
    Alex G. Larson and Donald Marcer

Communicating with Patients

IMPROVING COMMUNICATION, SATISFACTION AND COMPLIANCE

Philip Ley

London   Sydney   New York

CROOM HELM

First published in 1988 by Croom Helm Ltd
11 New Fetter Lane, London EC4P 4EE
Croom Helm Australia, 44–50 Waterloo Road,
North Ryde, 2113, New South Wales

Published in the USA by Croom Helm in association with
Chapman and Hall
29 West 35th Street, New York NY 10001

© 1988, Philip Ley

Typeset in 10/12pt Times by Leaper & Gard Ltd, Bristol
Printed in Great Britain at the University Press, Cambridge

ISBN 0 7099 4161 7 (Hb)
     0 7099 4174 9 (Pb)

British Library Cataloguing in Publication Data

Ley, Philip
    Communicating with patients.
    1. Medical personnel. Communication with patients.
    I. Title
    610.69'6

    ISBN 0–7099–4161–7 (hb)
         0–7099–4174–9 (pb)

Contents

Series Editor's Foreword

It is no exaggeration to say that throughout the first half of the twentieth century psychologists and doctors were seen as quite independent professionals, which if not openly hostile, had little to say to each other. Happily, the last two decades have seen a breaking down of these barriers as the two professions have come to recognise that they have much to learn from each other. This change in attitude is nowhere better illustrated than in the increasing part that the behavioural sciences have come to play in the training of doctors, nurses and other health professionals. Not surprisingly this shift of emphasis in medical education has been accompanied by a minor deluge of textbooks, all concerned with the relationship of psychology to medicine. Though many of these are excellent, the very depth of the subject matter that they seek to ecompass necessarily implies that many complex issues cannot be covered at other than a superficial level. Consequently, when I was asked by Croom Helm to produce such a text, I proposed instead a series under the general heading 'Psychology and Medicine'.

The series consists of individual texts, each dealing in some depth with a particular issue in which the two disciplines have a shared interest. Though most are written by psychologists with an established academic record, they are aimed primarily at practising professionals. Consequently the contributing authors have all had experience in teaching students or members of the medical and other health professions, and with very few exceptions have worked in a clinical setting. Thus they are well suited to fulfil the brief that is common to all the books in this series. That is, while the theoretical basis of the issue under discussion must be spelled out, it must be done in such a way that it enables readers (be they doctor, nurse, physiotherapist, etc. or student) to practise their professions more effectively.

Donald Marcer

Introduction

This book is concerned with the problem of how best to provide health related information to patients and clients. The literature on this subject has grown immensely over the last two decades and contributions to it have been made by members of most of the health care disciplines. Most of these contributions have reported the results of empirical research and it is with these that we shall be concerned. While the non-empirical contributions have contained many thoughtful and provocative ideas, at the end of the day the value of those ideas can only be assessed by experimental studies. The major exception to this generalisation is the literature concerning the ethical issues involved in providing information, and, in particular, the use of persuasive communications to increase patients' compliance with advice. Some reference to this will be made at various points in the text, but there will be no attempt to cover this literature in detail. The implicit stance of this book is that the provision of information to patients is desirable because, first, people want information about their illnesses and treatment, and secondly, because the provision of information has effects which are generally considered desirable.

Unfortunately there are problems in communicating effectively with patients. These include:

(a) making the information to be communicated comprehensible;
(b) finding ways to reduce the frequent forgetting which occurs;
(c) finding ways of encouraging feedback, and overcoming the diffidence that many people feel in clinical situations.

What is said by clinicians to patients is frequently not understood and frequently forgotten. It is probably worth emphasising at this point that although these problems are often referred to as 'failures' of patients' comprehension and memory, it is obvious that patients are not at fault. If a message is not understood by its intended audience, it is more rational, if blame must be attached at all, to blame the originator of the message for not making it comprehensible in the first place. With regard to forgetting, it is a matter of common observation that people forget much of what they are told. Not surprisingly, this has been confirmed in laboratory studies, and in real life studies, which have investigated a wide range of topics such as cocktail waitresses' memory for drinks orders, (Bennett, 1983); memory for weather forecasts and road traffic reports, (Wagenaar, 1978); and memory for news broadcasts, (Gunter, Berry and Clifford, 1982). It should not then be surprising that patients should forget some of what they are told. These problems of understanding, memory and diffidence account, in part, for patients frequently feeling dissatisfied with the communications aspect of their encounters with health care personnel, and also contribute to the high frequency with which health-related advice is not followed.

Amongst the possible solutions to this problem are the following:

(a) changing patients' behaviour;
(b) changing clinicians' behaviour;
(c) using additional supplementary means of communication.

While there have been some successful attempts to change patients' behaviour in clinical situations these have usually been expensive in terms of professionals' time. For example, Roter (1977) arranged for an experimental group of patients to be interviewed before their consultation. The aims of this interview were to elicit patients' expectations for information; to make the expectation for information salient; to provide an opportunity for the patient to rehearse questions prior to the encounter with the physician; to assist the patient in the articulation of the questions; and to encourage the patient actually to ask the questions by writing the questions down for the patient and providing support and approval for question asking. This procedure required about 15 minutes of skilled professional time. Incidentally, the results of this study were that both patients and physicians expressed more negative emotions in the consultation, but patients exposed to this intervention procedure were more likely to keep their next appointments. Thus, changing patients' behaviour is a possibility but it could be a costly exercise if attempted on a one to one basis. Presumably similar results could be obtained by mass educational methods or by the provision of written or audiovisual information in waiting areas.

In many ways attempting to change the clinicians' communicative behaviour would seem to be a more sensible strategy. If there are practicable ways of improving communication skills and techniques, then it should be relatively easy to incorporate these into educational programmes, or present them in books and journals. The main problems here are, as we shall see, first, that although techniques are available which can lead to worthwhile improvement they are by no means completely successful in overcoming the problems of understanding and memory, and secondly, just as patients are often non-compliant with advice so too are clinicians. Health care professionals do not always follow advice concerning better patient care. These two problems lead to the need to consider the use of supplementary aids to communication.

These supplementary aids have included the use of audiovisual presentations which the patient can view after the consultation, e.g. Midgeley and Macrae (1971), and providing the patient with a tape recording of the consultation, e.g. Butt (1977), but the commonest form of supplementary information provision is a leaflet, booklet, or other form of written material. As we shall see, there is good evidence that such written information can aid the communication process. It too has problems associated with it. It is often not noticed, often not read, frequently not understood, and often forgotten.

Fortunately it is possible to reduce professional non-compliance by providing information, feedback, and by the use of behavioural techniques. Interestingly enough these are the techniques which reduce patients' non-compliance. It is also possible to improve written information so as to increase the probability that it will be read, understood, and remembered.

The possible benefits of improved communication include:

(a) greater patient satisfaction;
(b) better patient cooperation with treatment regimens;
(c) reduced anxiety and distress;
(d) quicker recovery from surgery;
(e) shorter lengths of stay in hospital.

All of these are clearly worthwhile aims, and in these days of cost-efficiency it is worth noting that both better patient cooperation in treatment and shorter hospital stays can save a great deal of money. Thus improved communication can be justified not only in the human terms of greater satisfaction and reduced distress, but probably also in terms of hard cash.

Communication always takes place in a particular context, and not surprisingly there have been several investigations into the nature of the patient–clinician interaction. Some of these have been designed to derive a classification of such interactions. A good example of this sort of study is that of Byrne and Long (1976). These investigators undertook a content analysis of 2500 consultants and found clusters of physician behaviours which could be arranged on a patient-centred to physician-centred continuum. Thus they describe four diagnostic styles ranging from the most patient-centred ones of high use of listening, reflecting and silence, and high use of clarifying and interpretation, to the physician-centred styles of high use of analysing and probing and active information-gathering. Similarly the seven prescriptive styles found could be arranged along the same continuum. These ranged from the physician allowing the patient to make decisions at the patient-centred end to the physician making all the decisions and giving the patient non-debatable instructions at the physician-centred end. Byrne and Long also reported that these styles tended to be invariant across patients.

Other investigators have conducted micro-analyses of linguistic and other interactions in the consultation, e.g. Litton-Hawes (1978), Frankel (1980). Litton-Hawes analysed 16 consultations to derive the rules which governed who should speak and what they should speak about. An example of such a rule is as follows. If the physician asks about a topic, the patient may ask a question about that topic before answering the physician's question. Frankel similarly studied the minutiae of the interaction and discovered regularities in behaviour such as the physician, just prior to touching the patient's body in a physical examination, starting to talk about something unrelated to the problem. Studies such as these, because they require so much time for their analysis, are inevitably based on small samples of physicians and patients which of course raises the question of the generality of their findings.

To date it is probably fair to say that these approaches to the context in which the communication occurs have not yielded effective techniques for improving communication. For this reason they will not be reviewed in detail, but where aspects of the interaction are related to outcomes of interest, as for example in the studies of Korsch, Gozzi and Francis (1968) or Larsen and Smith (1981), they will of course be mentioned.

Despite the attention that they have received over the past two decades or so, (Davis, 1966; Ley and Spelman, 1967; Fletcher, 1973; Bennett, 1976; Sackett and Haynes, 1976; Haynes, Taylor, and Sackett, 1979; DiMatteo and DiNicola, 1982; Pendleton and Hasler, 1983), there is no evidence that the problems of patients' dissatisfaction with communications and their often low cooperation in treatment are diminishing. This is one of the reasons why reference has been freely made to studies conducted some years ago. For example, the earliest investigation of patients' satisfaction with communications cited is 1961, (the latest being 1985). Year of publication is not related to percentage reported as being satisfied with communications ($r = -0.12$). The second reason for including some early studies is forcibly to remind the reader that these problems are longstanding ones which show no signs of spontaneous remission.

Some attention is given to the methodological problems involved in investigation of the topics covered. This is desirable in order for the reader to appreciate better the status of some of the evidence reviewed, and because, as in many other fields, there is still a great deal of research needed. Indeed it is hoped that some readers at least will be tempted into research on these topics. However, as the book is intended for practitioners and students as well as researchers, an attempt has been made throughout and in a summary chapter to spell out the practical implications of the research reviewed. Finally, because it is possible that not all readers will be familiar with some of the statistical terms used a brief glossary of these terms is appended to this Introduction.

Glossary

correlation coefficient
: is an index of the degree of relationship between two variables, e.g. patient satisfaction and compliance, which normally ranges between between zero and one. Higher values indicate a stronger relationship. It is positive when high scores on one variable are associated with high scores on the other variable, and negative, when high scores on one are associated with low scores on the other.

effect size
: is a value used in meta-analysis. Its usual formula is:
(Mean of treated group − mean of control group)/Standard deviation of control group.
The formula yields a value, which for any study, gives the difference between means of the treated and control groups as a number of control group standard deviation units. This permits comparisons to be made across studies which have used different outcome measures.

eta coefficient
: is very similar to a correlation coefficient.

meta-analysis
: refers to a set of techniques for providing a quantitative summary or review of studies, even when they have used different outcome measures.

multiple correlation coefficient
: is an index which expresses the degree of relationship between two or more predictor variables (considered simultaneously) and a criterion,

	e.g. the relationship between understanding, memory, and satisfaction taken as a group (predictor variables) and compliance (criterion). The coefficient ranges between zero and one. Higher values indicate a stronger relationship.
p	is the probability that a finding is due to chance. Probabilities range between zero and one. It is conventional to label a finding as 'statistically significant' if the probability of its occurring by chance is less than 0.05 (less than 5 chances in 100). Other levels commonly reported are $p<0.01$, and $p<0.001$.
Phi coefficient	is a type of correlation coefficient.
significance, statistical	*see 'p'.*
standard deviation	is a measure of dispersion or spread of values or scores.
Tau coefficient	is a type of correlation coefficient.

1

Patients' Satisfaction

INTRODUCTION

Patients' levels of satisfaction with various aspects of the care they receive are important for two main reasons. The first of these is that patient satisfaction is a desirable goal in its own right. The second, as we shall see, is that patient satisfaction is an important determinant of patients' compliance with advice.

Studies of people's satisfaction with the various aspects of health care have been of two main types. Some investigations have attempted to assess satisfaction with health care in general, i.e. unrelated to a specific episode or illness, others have been concerned with satisfaction in relation to particular encounters or sets of encounters with health care personnel. These latter studies have used as their samples subjects who were currently or who had recently been patients.

In the context of our present concerns it is patients' satisfaction with the communications aspect of their clinical interactions which is of interest. However, it will be useful to describe some of the research on the relationships between satisfaction with communications and satisfaction with other aspects of the consultation.

THE MEASUREMENT OF SATISFACTION

Investigations of patients' satisfaction have used a range of interview and questionnaire measures differing tremendously in level of methodological sophistication.

The simplest method of all has been to use a general question about the area or areas which are of interest. This technique has been used in a number of studies. Examples of such questions are:

> While you were in hospital were you able to find out all you wanted to know about your condition, your treatment, and your progress or not? (Parkin, 1976)
>
> Looking at things as a whole, how satisfied are you with the medical care that you receive? (Department of Defense, 1975)

Almost as simple has been the use of a number of separate questions about different aspects of care.

> Have you been told enough about what is wrong with you?
> Have you been told enough about your progress?
> Have you been told enough about the treatment?
> Have you been told enough about the results of investigations?
> (Spelman, Ley and Jones, 1966)

The use of a number of separate questions has also sometimes been accompanied by multiple choice answers so that a satisfaction score can be derived. A satisfaction score is often desirable because it has a number of advantages for statistical purposes. The following examples are drawn from DiMatteo, Prince, and Taranta (1978), (the numbers in parentheses are the scores awarded to the specified answer):

> 'Does the doctor explain your medical condition to you so that:
>
> you understand it perfectly (3);
> or only a little (2);
> or not explain anything at all (1)?
>
> Does the doctor ever ask about your family?
> No (0);
> Yes (1).'

Ley and his colleagues, e.g. Ley, Bradshaw, Kincey and Atherton (1976a); Ley, Whitworth, Skilbeck, Woodward, Pinsent, Pike, Clarkson and Clark (1976b), have utilised a technique which also falls into this category. The questions used have had the following format:

Did you want to know about the results of tests and investigations?
If so, were you told:

(a) enough
(b) not enough
(c) nothing

The questions could be presented either orally or in written form, and covered a number of topics. A satisfaction score was derived by assigning a score of 2, 1 or 0 to the answers 'enough', 'not enough' and 'nothing' respectively for each of the topics where the patient had stated that they wanted information. These scores were summed and this total was divided by 2 times the number of topics on which the patient wanted information. This yielded a score which was a proportion of the maximum possible score for that patient.

Other investigators have favoured the use of a Likert-type format for their questionnaire. This consists of presenting the subject with a number of statements and asking the subject to indicate the extent to which they agree or disagree with the statement. The possible responses being: 'strongly agree'; 'agree'; 'uncertain'; 'disagree'; and 'strongly disagree'. The responses are scored from 1 to 5 for each item, and summed to form a total satisfaction score, covering a number of aspects of satisfaction with the consultation or medical care. In the proper versions of the Likert method each item appearing in the final scale is there because preliminary investigations have shown that it has a high correlation with total score. However, some questionnaires which have adopted the format have omitted this important step.

Typical examples of items are:

The doctor told me all I wanted to know about my illness.
The doctor really gave me a chance to say what was on my mind.
The doctor gave me a thorough check-up.
(Wolf, Putnam, James, and Stiles, 1978)

I felt my feelings and concerns were considered when recommendations were made.
The doctor gave me a clear indication of how to take the medication.
(Falvo, Woehlke and Deichmann, 1980).

Another traditional attitude scale construction technique, the Thurstone method, has also been used. In this technique judges are asked to rate each of a large pool of items on an 11 point scale for degree of favourableness towards the object being judged. The mean (or median) rating awarded by the judges to each item is then calculated, and a measure of the spread of judges' ratings for each item is also calculated. This last measure is then used to reject items on which the judges show too much disagreement. From the remainder items are then selected so that the final scale consists of items covering the whole range of favourableness in terms of the mean values awarded by the judges. Each item has a scale value which is the mean rating awarded by the judges. Scores on the final scale consist of either the sum or the mean of the items with which the subject expresses agreement. The sum or the mean of the values of the items selected is used if the subject has to respond to a stated number of items, e.g. the three which come nearest to express-ing their opinion, while the mean is used if subjects have a free choice about how many items to respond to. This technique has been used by Hulka and her associates, e.g. Hulka, Kupper, Daly, Cassel and Schoen (1975d) in modified form in that a Likert format, ('strongly agree' 'agree', etc.), was used as well, and scores were the product of the Likert score for the item weighted by the Thustone scale value of the item. Items used are similar to those given as examples of Likert scale items.

Finally much more sophisticated multivariate statistical methods, such as factor analysis, e.g. Ware and Snyder (1975), and multi-dimensional scaling, e.g. Roghmann, Hengst and Zastowny (1979), have been used in the construction of scales for measuring patient satisfaction.

THE SUBTYPES OF PATIENT SATISFACTION

Different investigators have concentrated on different aspects of patients' satisfaction. Ley and his collaborators have concen-trated their efforts on patients' satisfaction with communi-cations, which they have defined as patients' satisfaction with the quality and quantity of information they receive in the clinical encounter, e.g. Ley and Spelman (1967). Korsch and her colleagues have been concerned with a rating of patients' satisfaction with the clinical encounter as a whole, e.g. Korsch *et al.* (1968). Hulka and her colleagues have been concerned with three aspects of patients' satisfaction. These are (a) the professional competence of the physician; (b) the personal qualities of the physician; and (c) the costs and convenience of care, e.g. Hulka *et al.* (1975). Ware and associates, on the basis of their factor-analytic studies, have been concerned with four main dimensions of patients' attitudes. These are physician conduct; availability of services such as hospitals and specialists; continuity/convenience of care; and access mechanisms, e.g. Ware and Snyder (1975). Finally, Wolf *et al.* (1978) have developed the Medical Interview Satisfaction Scale, which measures three aspects of the doctor–patient encounter. These are satisfaction with (a) the cognitive aspect, which is essentially a measure of satisfaction with the amount and quality of the information provided by the doctor; (b) the affective aspect, which is a measure of the extent to which the patient feels that the doctor listens, understands, and is interested; and (c) the behavioural aspect, which is concerned with the patient's evaluation of the doctor's competence in the consultation.

There is some evidence available on the relationships between different aspects of patients' satisfaction with the medical encounter. Korsch *et al.* (1968) provided data on the relationships between the patients' perception of (a) the doctor as a good communicator, (b) the doctor being able to understand, and an overall rating of patients' satisfaction. The first of these is obviously a measure of satisfaction with communications in the sense used by Ley, and the second is related to what Wolf *et al.* (1978) have termed satisfaction with the affective aspect of consultations.

Ware and Snyder (1975) and Doyle and Ware (1977) reported the correlation of their subscale 'Information-giving/ explanation', which is a measure of satisfaction with communications, and their Satisfaction with Physician Conduct factor. This factor provides an overall measure of satisfaction with the medical encounter.

DiMatteo, Prince and Taranta (1978) used a number of questions of interest in their measure of satisfaction. One of these can clearly be taken as a measure of satisfaction with communications:

Does the doctor explain your medical condition to you so that you understand it?

5

Two other questions are clearly related to the affective aspect of the consultation:

Does the doctor listen to what you say?
Do you think the doctor cares for you as a person?

Finally two further questions seem to be related to what is measured by the Behavioral Scale of Wolf *et al.*

Do you feel the doctor spent enough time with you?
Do you think your doctor is not as smart as other doctors?

Wolf *et al.* (1978) presented data on the relationships between the individual items and their satisfaction scales, and the overall satisfaction score. One of these items was:

The doctor told me all I wanted to know about my illness.

This can clearly be taken as a measure of satisfaction with communications, as can their cognitive scale as a whole.

Table 1.1 provides a summary of these data. It should be

Table 1.1: Relationships between different measures of patient satisfaction

Aspect of satisfaction	Correlation with aspect of satisfaction		
	General	Behavioural	Affective
Satisfaction with communication			
Korsch *et al.* (1968)	0.54	—	—
Ware and Snyder (1975)	0.70	—	—
Doyle and Ware (1977)	0.64	—	—
DiMatteo *et al.* (1978)	—	0.25 (time)	0.39 (listens)
		0.22 (smart)	0.27 (cares)
Wolf *et al.* (1978)			
(a) question	0.71	0.56	0.66
(b) Cognitive Scale	—	0.62	0.75
Satisfaction with the affective features of the interaction			
Korsch *et al.* (1968)	0.38	—	—
DiMatteo *et al.* (1978)			
(a) listens	—	0.28 (time)	—
	—	0.14 (smart)	
(b) cares	—	0.18 (time)	—
	—	0.23 (smart)	—
Wolf *et al.* (1978)	—	0.76	—

noted that as the correlations given for Korsch *et al.* and DiMatteo *et al.* are Phi and Tau coefficients these would be expected to have smaller numerical values than the other correlations in the table. This effect will be further exaggerated by the fact that these correlations involve single items.

It would appear from this evidence that measures of satisfaction with communications have reasonably high correlations with measures of (a) satisfaction with the doctor–patient interaction as a whole, and (b) satisfaction with other aspects of the consultation. Before describing research into patients' satisfaction in more detail it is worth considering some of the correlates of satisfaction with the consultation as a whole.

CORRELATES OF SATISFACTION WITH THE CONSULTATION

A great deal of the evidence available on this topic comes from the major study of 800 consultations in a paediatric clinic by Korsch *et al.* (1968). These investigators reported that satisfaction with the consultation as a whole was associated with:

(a) The doctor being friendly rather than businesslike;
(b) The doctor being seen as understanding the patients' concerns;
(c) Patients' expectations about treatment and the like being met;
(d) The doctor being perceived as a good communicator;
(e) The provision of information.

In this investigation length of time spent with the physician was not related to patients' satisfaction, although other investigators have found such a relationship, e.g. Smith, Polis, and Hadac (1981). In this last study it was also found that the provision of information by the physician was also associated with patient satisfaction. This finding echoes that of Bertakis (1977) who reported that the greater the amount of information given by the physician, the greater was the patient's satisfaction.

Stiles, Putnam, Wolf and James (1979) reported that while affective satisfaction (see above for definition), was associated with the amount of time spent in the patient giving information to the doctor (explaining their problem in their own words),

7

cognitive satisfaction was related to the amount of time that the physician spent giving the patient information.

Stiles *et al.* utilised a quite complicated system for coding the interactions between patients and physicians, and other investigators have also used sophisticated systems. The main ones in use currently are those of Bales (1950), Roter (1977) (a modification of the Bales system) and the system of Stiles and co-workers, Stiles (1978), Stiles *et al.* (1979). In a comparative study of these systems, Inui, Carter, Kukull, and Haigh (1982), found that the Bales system and Roter's modification thereof were better at predicting patient satisfaction than the Stiles' system.

Other investigators have explored the relationship between non-verbal communication and patient satisfaction. For example, Larsen and Smith (1981) used the classification of non-verbal communication devised by Mehrabian (1972) to analyse 34 patient–physician consultations. This system measures three main categories of non-verbal behaviour. The first is 'immediacy', which is the degree of 'closeness' between the participants. This is assessed from frequency of touching, eye contact, leaning forward, body orientation, and physical proximity. The second category is 'relaxation'. This is assessed from observations of the degree of relaxation of hand and neck, the degree of asymmetry in arm and leg positions, and the amount of sideways or backward leaning. The third category is 'responsiveness'. This is assessed from facial activity, vocal activity, speech rate, and speech volume. Larsen and Smith found that the overall rating of physician immediacy was related to patients' levels of satisfaction, as were three of the submeasures of immediacy (touching, forward leaning, and body orientation). In addition two of the relaxation submeasures (backward leaning and neck relaxation), were related to satisfaction. It is likely that there will be much further research into the effects of patient–physician interaction in both its verbal and non-verbal modes.

Finally as we shall see shortly, patients' satisfaction is related to their understanding and recall of what they are told.

PATIENTS' SATISFACTION WITH COMMUNICATIONS

There is a large amount of evidence available to show that patients are frequently dissatisfied with the quality and amount of information they receive from medical and other hospital staff, and from their general practitioners. Patients feel that they have not been given enough information. Data from a number of studies of this topic are summarised in Table 1.2.

The median per cent dissatisfied for the hospital samples is 38; for the general practice and community samples is 26 per cent; and for psychiatric patients 39 per cent. Further, as noted in the Introduction, the date of the survey is unrelated to the percentage reporting dissatisfaction.

SOME COMPLICATING FACTORS

A number of factors would be expected to affect the percentages reporting themselves as satisfied with communications. For example studies using as their base the first encounter of an illness episode, and asking detailed questions (Kincey, Bradshaw and Ley 1975; Ley et al., 1975; 1976b) reported higher levels of dissatisfaction in general practice patients than the study which asked a general question about communications not related to a specific episode (Kaim-Caudle and Marsh, 1975), and the study which asked a general question about a particular episode (Cartwright, 1983). In addition there will be variation associated with the different doctors involved as communicators, and the types of patients studied. However, there were also some puzzling features of the earlier data.

In the case of studies of hospital patients Ley (1972a) noted that, across the various samples, there seemed to be a curvilinear relationship between the percentage of patients reporting satisfaction and the time elapsing since discharge from hospital. Higher satisfaction was reported in studies which followed up patients in the week or so immediately after discharge; low satisfaction in those with a two to four week follow-up; and higher satisfaction again in those with a follow-up of eight weeks or more. Ley et al. (1976a) confirmed this relationship within a sample of discharged medical patients, and found higher satisfaction amongst patients interviewed one or eight weeks after discharge than amongst those interviewed at two or four weeks. Unfortunately there are mixed findings here in that Spelman et al. (1966) reported that satisfaction with communications increased with increasing time since discharge.

Ley (1972a) also noted that in some of the studies he

9

Table 1.2: Results of surveys of patients' satisfaction with communications

Investigation	Type of patients	Percentage dissatisfied
(a) Hospital patients		
McGhie (1961)	490 medical and surgical	65
Hetherington *et al.* (1963)	80 medical	54
Cartwright (1964)	701 mixed	29
Hugh-Jones *et al.* (1964)	275 medical	39
Houghton (1968)	551 obstetric	35
Raphael (1969)	1348 mixed	18
Kennell *et al.* (1969)	60 pediatric	58
United Manchester Hospitals (1970)	811 mixed	5–17
Fisher (1971)	150 medical	22
Jolly *et al.* (1971)	113 obstetric	39
DeCastro (1972)	pediatric	8
Geersten *et al.* (1973)	123 arthritis	18
Ley *et al.* (1974)	80 surgical	23
Ley *et al.* (1976)	43 medical	53
Mayou *et al.* (1976)	40 coronary	
	(a) in hospital	82
	(b) after discharge	65
Parkin (1976)	134 medical	57
Hospital Affiliates (1978)	1053 national sample (USA)	32–51
Reynolds (1978)	100 surgical	55
Klein (1979)	788 mixed	32
Jones *et al.* (1982)	122 cancer	66
Meyerovitz *et al.* (1983)	57 cancer	33
(b) General practice and community		
Arnhold *et al.* (1970)	60 pediatric	32
Kaim-Caudle and Marsh (1975)	340 general practice	5–15
Kincey *et al.* (1975)	61 general practice	26
Ley *et al.* (1975)	70 general practice	37
Ley *et al.* (1976)	157 general practice	35
Baksas and Helgeland (1980)[a]	787 hypertensive	58
Berry *et al.* (1981)[a]	236 patients prescribed flurazepam	22
Kanouse *et al.* (1981)[a]	518 patients prescribed oestrogens	16
Winkler *et al.* (1981)[a]	793 patients prescribed erhythromycin	42
Cartwright (1983)	583 general practice	20
Sanazaro (1985)	201 with chronic condition	11
(c) Psychiatric patients		
Raphael and Peers (1972)	9 samples of psychiatric patients drawn from 9 different hospitals:	
	Median	39
	Range	31–54

a. satisfaction with information about treatment

reviewed the doctors involved were making special efforts to communicate information to patients, (Hugh-Jones, Tanser and Whitley, 1964; Hetherington, Ley, Spelman and Jones 1963; Houghton, 1968). In these studies satisfaction rates were no higher than in studies where no such special efforts were made. Further, although there had been a decade of interest and publicity about the problem, satisfaction rates recorded in studies conducted at later dates were no higher than those conducted at earlier dates. We have already noted that this still seems to be true as can be seen from Table 1.2. Also relevant is the finding of Ley *et al.* (1976b) who reported data on a sample of patients seen in the same hospital as those investigated earlier by Hetherington *et al.* (1963). The dissatisfaction rates were 53 and 54 per cent respectively despite there being a time gap of nine years between the dates of data collection.

A further finding was that there seemed to be little if any relationship between whether patients reported that they had been given information in hospital and their satisfaction with communications (Spelman, Ley and Jones, 1966; Ley and Spelman, 1967).

To summarise:

(a) When doctors feel they are making special efforts satisfaction rates seem to be no higher;
(b) Patients who report that they have been told about their illnesses, treatment, investigations, etc., are no less likely to be dissatisfied;
(c) Despite a considerable emphasis on the importance of good communication in medical education, and in the professional literature there is no evidence that dissatisfaction rates are dropping.

A number of hypotheses could possibly explain the finding that the provision of information did not seem to reduce dissatisfaction with communications.

The first of these was that dissatisfaction with communications was merely a reflection of more general dissatisfaction. Thus, factors which affected communications would only result in greater satisfaction in that particular area if they also reduced dissatisfaction in general. The obvious prediction from this hypothesis is that dissatisfaction with other areas of medical and nursing care should parallel dissatisfaction with communications.

11

This does not seem to be so. Satisfaction with other aspects of care seems to be considerably higher (Ley, 1972a; Lebow, 1976; Mayou, Williamson and Foster, 1976; Hospital Affiliates International, 1978).

A second possibility is that patients of a certain personality want something to complain about and seize on the area of communications because it is more nebulous than other areas. Presumably this would lead us to expect that patients who complain about poor communications will differ in personality from those who do not complain. Ley (1976) investigated this hypothesis by administering the Cattell Sixteen Personality Factor Questionnaire to a group of patients who were satisfied with communications and a group who were not. The groups did not differ significantly on any of the first or second order factors measured by the test. However, Spelman *et al.* (1966) found that patients who reported feeling depressed while in hospital were significantly more likely to be dissatisfied with communications than those who did not. In the group reporting depression the dissatisfaction rate was 79 per cent, while for the group not reporting depression it was 36 per cent. This finding presents some difficulties of interpretation in that it is possible that the depressed patients were depressed because of lack of information. This interpretation cannot be made of the results reported by Ley (1976) who measured depression using the Hildreth Feeling Scale (Hildreth, 1946) and found that, as in the case of dissatisfaction with communications there was an inverted 'U' relationship with time since discharge, depression being lower at 1 and 8 weeks than at 2 or 4 weeks. Unfortunately no correlation between depression and dissatisfaction was calculated. These results therefore suggest that there is probably no relationship between personality and dissatisfaction, but that some significant relationship with mood might exist.

The third hypothesis is that increased information giving is ineffective because patients often do not understand what they are told, and often do not remember what they are told. These factors, combined with patients' diffidence about asking for information when they are not sure what is meant, or when they want more information, have two main consequences. First, even in situations where clinicians wish to provide full information they will not be successful in improving communications because what they say is often not in understandable or memorable form. Secondly, because patients do not provide feedback in the form of questions, clinicians remain unaware of their faults in communicating. These factors will be discussed in detail in the next two chapters.

SUMMARY

The main points of this chapter can be summarised as follows.

(a) Satisfaction with communications aspect of the consultation correlates highly with satisfaction with other aspects of the clinician–patient interaction.

(b) Substantial numbers of patients feel dissatisfied with the communications aspect of their clinical encounters. This contrasts with usually high levels of satisfaction with other aspects of the clinician–patient interaction.

(c) This dissatisfaction does not seem to be reduced by clinicians trying (in untutored ways), to see that patients are fully informed. Nor does the increase in the level of educational and research concern with the problem over the last two decades seem to have led to a reduction in patients' dissatisfaction.

(d) In addition there is evidence that patients who say that they have been told about various aspects of their condition are just as likely to be dissatisfied as those who say they have not.

(e) It is likely that telling patients is in itself not enough. They have to be told in ways that they can understand and remember. Because of lack of feedback in the form of questions and comments it is difficult for clinicians to improve their performance as communicators.

2

Patients' Understanding of What They are Told

INTRODUCTION

It is likely that patients will not understand and will misinterpret much of what they are told. There are two main reasons for these failures in comprehension. The first is that clinicians often present information to patients in too difficult a form. The second is that patients often have their own theories about illnesses and naturally enough interpret new information within the framework of their existing ideas. Where the patients' ideas are discrepant from those of the clinician it is likely that the message received will often not be the one intended.

Examples of the use of language which is too difficult have appeared frequently in the literature. For example, Korsch, Gozzi and Francis (1968), and Korsch and Negrete (1972) reported that doctors in a paediatric clinic were using terms such as 'labia', 'sphincter', 'incubation period', 'nares', 'peristalsis', 'Coombs titre' and 'lumbar puncture', without explanation. These terms were often not understood or were misinterpreted. For example, some thought that a lumbar puncture was an operation to drain the lungs, and some that the incubation period was the time the child would have to stay in bed.

Examples of patients' theories which might cause difficulties in understanding the information presented by clinicians also abound in the literature. A good example is the study of Roth, Caron, Ort, Berger, Merrill, Albee and Streeter (1962) of patients' beliefs about peptic ulcer and its treatment. Many patients thought that acid caused ulcers, but only 10 per cent had a reasonably clear idea that acid is secreted by the stomach. Many thought that acid was introduced into the stomach in food that was eaten or came from the teeth when food was chewed. At that time it was almost universal for patients with duodenal ulcer to be instructed to eat small frequent meals. It is easy to imagine the confusion caused by such an instruction in the minds of those patients who believed that (a) ulcers are caused by too much acid; and (b) that acid gets into the stomach when food is chewed or eaten. To these patients the advice about eating small frequent meals would have amounted to an instruction to increase the amount of acid in their stomachs and thus, on the face of it, make their ulcers worse.

Obviously many of these misunderstandings could be cleared up if patients would ask questions when they did not understand the language used or when statements were made which seemed to conflict with what they knew or thought they knew. Unfortunately patients seem very reluctant to ask questions in clinical situations.

PATIENTS' RELUCTANCE TO ASK QUESTIONS

The fact that patients are often very diffident about seeking information has been noted by several reviewers (Central Health Services Council, 1963; Cartwright, 1964; Ley and Spelman, 1967; Ley, 1972a; Roter, 1977, 1983). Some researchers have studied the proportion of patients asking questions. Mayou *et al.* (1976) found that 70 per cent of their coronary inpatients did not intend to ask questions about their condition even though many of them wanted more information, and in a study of general practice patients Boreham and Gibson (1978) found that the vast majority of their patients asked no questions about significant areas of diagnosis or treatment about which they had not been informed. For example, 37 per cent of these patients were given no clear instructions for treatment, and none of these asked any questions about this topic.

These studies of the percentages of patients asking questions beg the question of whether all of the patients involved wanted more information or not. Fortunately, some investigations have provided data concerning patients who did want to know, and who nevertheless failed to ask questions. Korsch *et al.* (1968) found that 24 per cent of the parents of the pediatric patients in their study did not ask the doctor questions even though they wanted more information. In addition these investigators found

15

that 76 per cent of the parents' main worries and 63 per cent of their expectations about treatment were not communicated to the physician. Carstairs (1970) reported that 53 per cent of patients who wanted more information failed to ask for it. The patients were a random sample of patients in hospitals in Scotland. Fisher (1971) found that 11 per cent of a mixed out-patient sample would not ask for the information which they required. A higher percentage of reluctance to ask questions was discovered by Ley, Skilbeck, and Tulips (1975), who found that 27 per cent of patients reported that although they usually wanted more information when they consulted their doctor they never asked questions. Further, patients interviewed just after their latest consultation were asked whether they had asked for more information in different areas where they wanted it. The percentages who had wished for information in these different areas but not asked for it were: for diagnosis 42 per cent; for treatment 41 per cent; for other advice 75 per cent. Klein (1979), summarising a large-scale British survey, reported that almost half those who wanted to make requests for further information had failed to do so.

This reluctance to ask questions probably stems mainly from over-deferential attitudes towards doctors. Its main consequences are (a) patients being less informed about their condition than they would like, (b) absence of feedback to clinicians about the adequacy of their performance as communicators, and (c) clinicians believing that patients do not want information.

PATIENTS' UNDERSTANDING OF MEDICAL TERMINOLOGY

It is probably worth noting immediately that, as Mazzullo, Lasagna and Griner (1974) have pointed out, even simple everyday words can be ambiguous in a medical context. The example they give is the word 'for'. A tablet taken 'for pain' reduces pain. However a tablet taken 'for sleeping' does not reduce it, it causes it. What then do people think if the tablet is 'for fluid retention'? Such tablets are of course intended to reduce fluid retention, but Mazzullo *et al.* found that 52 per cent of their sample thought that the tablet would cause fluid retention. These investigators point out that this could lead to patients taking the tablet in entirely the wrong fashion, avoiding it when they notice symptoms of oedema. The moral is clear. Avoid ambiguity. The problem is of course to notice its existence.

Several investigators have devised tests of understanding of medical vocabulary which they have then administered to samples of patients or of people in general. Some of these were reviewed by Ley and Spelman (1967) and included the investigation by Redlich (1949) which asked patients for the definition of 60 medical terms. Not surprisingly Redlich found considerable variation in the percentage who could define the different words in the list. The percentages understanding the terms 'infection', 'cancer', 'lesion', 'prognosis', 'metastasis' were 96, 90, 24, 4, and 0 per cent respectively.

Later researchers have also used tests of patients' understanding of medical terminology. Boyle (1970), using a multiple choice test, assessed patients' understanding of the terms: 'arthritis', 'heartburn', 'jaundice', 'palpitation', 'bronchitis', 'piles', and 'flatulence'. He found that the percentages giving the correct definition were 86, 85, 77, 52, 80, 74, and 43 per cent respectively. Boyle also investigated patients' knowledge of the anatomical location of major organs of the body. Once more a multiple choice test was used. This consisted of outlines of the human body each containing a shaded area. The test questions consisted of presenting the subject with four such outlines, in one of which the shaded area corresponded to the location of the organ whose location the patient was being asked to identify. Using this technique Boyle found that 42 per cent of patients knew the location of the heart; 60 per cent the bladder; 46 per cent the kidneys; 20 per cent the stomach; 51 per cent the lungs; 77 per cent the intestines; 49 per cent the liver; and 70 per cent the thyroid gland.

Tring and Hayes-Allen (1973) administered Boyle's multiple choice test of understanding of terminology to medical and dental undergraduates and to postgraduate students of education. The percentages giving the correct definitions of 'arthritis', 'heartburn', 'jaundice', 'palpitation', 'bronchitis', 'piles', and 'flatulence' were 82, 88, 61, 68, 80, 83, and 51 respectively. These figures are quite close to those of Boyle's patients and show that with vocabulary items such as these, better-educated groups can also have problems.

Another example is the investigation by Cole (1979), who

used a multiple choice questionnaire to assess the understand-ability of words appearing in health education materials. The sample studied consisted of 60 general practice patients and 60 polytechnic students. Over half the sample did not under-stand the terms 'dilated', 'antiemetics', 'haemorrhoids', and a third or more did not understand 'abdomen', 'emaciation', or 'endemic'.

A further example comes from the report of the Adult Liter-acy Support Services Fund (1980). The samples studied included students of English as a second language, and adults with reading difficulties attending Adult Literacy classes. Words which provided particular difficulty for these groups included 'weaning', 'nourishment', 'alkaline', 'symptoms', 'directed', 'persist' and 'inhale'. Statements which were very difficult for these groups included:

'unless otherwise directed by the doctor'
'Do not exceed the stated dose'
'Consult your doctor if symptoms persist'.

In a slightly different context Ley, Flaherty, Smith, Martin and Renner (1985) investigated the problem of how well high school students and adults understood the words used in two warning labels. Two warning labels were studied. The first was: 'Intentional misuse by deliberately concentrating and inhaling contents can be harmful or fatal'; and the second: 'Do not deliberately sniff this product. Sniffing might harm or kill you'. Over 90 per cent of the adult sample could define the words and phrases adequately except for 'concentrating' and 'deliber-ately concentrating'. In contrast the high school students had great difficulty with many of the words. Thus 'fatal' was under-stood by only 48 per cent; 'misuse' by 35 per cent; 'inhaling' by 75 per cent; 'concentrating' by 6 per cent; 'contents' by 56 per cent; 'product' by 73 per cent; and 'harmful' by 70 per cent. As the warnings in this case were primarily aimed at high school students it is clear that simpler vocabulary should have been used. Note also that the words used are likely to occur in a variety of clinical contexts.

Results such as those just described have to be interpreted with caution. The samples used have not been chosen in such a way as to guarantee that they are representative of the popu-lation at large. The results of multiple choice tests depend partly on the exact details of the question, especially the alternative wrong answers provided. Further, it would be expected, with the amount of media attention given to medical and health topics, that levels of knowledge in the general population might be constantly rising. Nevertheless at the time that each of the studies just described was conducted it was considered reasonable that most patients would be expected to understand the terms in question. They are used by clinicians in their communications to patients, or, in the study by Cole, were in use in health education materials, and in the study by Ley *et al.* the words were drawn from warning labels in current use. It therefore seems safe to conclude that there is at least some risk of people being presented with words whose meaning they do not know in a variety of health related settings.

PATIENTS' KNOWLEDGE OF COMMON DISEASES

A number of investigators have inquired into general levels of knowledge about particular illnesses. As is true of studies of understanding of medical terminology it would be expected that the results of such investigations will be heavily time and culture bound. Some of these studies have had as their aim the discovery of common misconceptions which could affect the success of doctor–patient communication. Ley and Spelman (1967) conducted an investigation of this kind and found some relatively common misconceptions. Thus 28 per cent did not associate coronary thrombosis with the heart, and 44 per cent of their sample did not know that the prognosis in lung cancer was as gloomy as it is. Indeed 20 per cent thought that lung cancer was easily cured. Further it was shown by Spelman and Ley (1966) that the seriousness of the prognosis was less appreciated by heavy smokers than by others. In similar vein Leventhal, Meyer, and Nerentz (1980) reported misconceptions about their illness amongst hypertensive patients. Nearly a third thought that hypertension was an illness likely to be cured by short-term treatment.

Other investigators have been concerned with discovering misconceptions and levels of knowledge about a particular disease or subset of diseases with a view to developing educational programmes for patients suffering from the particular disorder. A good example of this approach is the programme of research into peptic ulcer reported by Roth *et al.* (1962), Caron and Roth (1977) and Roth (1979). The finding that several patients did not realise that acid is secreted by the stomach has already been mentioned and has obvious implications for the design of educational material for such patients.

There is probably little point in further description of such studies. Suffice to say that they show that misconceptions are not uncommon and that patients often lack basic background knowledge that their clinicians assume them to have. (Recall the examples given earlier from the investigations by Korsch and her collaborators.) All of this must lead to the prediction that in the ordinary clinical situation patients will often fail to understand what they are told.

Assessment of patients' understanding of what they have been told in their clinical encounters has been carried out by three main methods. The first of these is the patient's own report of whether they have understood or not. The second method is for the patient to be interviewed by an expert who then makes an assessment of how well the patient has understood. The third method, used in the case of instructions and advice is the quasi-behavioural test which asks the patient questions about what they would do when attempting to follow the advice. Results obtained by all of these methods suggest that failures to understand are not infrequent.

UNDERSTANDING AS ASSESSED BY THE PATIENTS' OWN REPORTS

In three studies of general practice patients Ley and his collaborators have asked patients whether they understood what they were told about various aspects of their illnesses. Patients were making their first attendance with an illness from which they had not previously suffered. The results of these investigations are summarised in Table 2.1. It can be seen that these general practice patients frequently felt that they had not understood what they had been told. Other studies in other types of setting also report that patients have complained of not understanding (e.g. Korsch, Freeman and Negrete, 1971).

One of the problems with the use of patients' own reports as a measure of understanding is of course the possibility that the patient will think that they have understood when in fact they

Table 2.1: Patients' reports of not understanding what they have been told

	Percentage *not* understanding what they were told about:			
Investigation	Diagnosis	Aetiology	Treatment	Prognosis
Kincey *et al.* (1975)	7	17	14	13
Ley *et al.* (1975)	47	47	43	53
Ley *et al.* (1976)	(a)30	43	—	35
	(b)34	40	—	35

have not. It would therefore be expected that this method would tend to underestimate failures to understand.

PATIENTS' UNDERSTANDING AS ASSESSED BY EXPERT JUDGES

The second method of assessing patients' understanding is the use of expert judges. Most of this research seems to have been concerned with patients' understanding of treatment advice, particularly understanding of medication regimens. It is likely that many of these investigations have used as their criterion of understanding the patients' ability to repeat or paraphrase the treatment advice. The difficulty here is that the patients' inter-pretation may not be the same as the investigators. Thus suppose a patient on a diuretic was asked what the purpose of the medication was, and replied that it was 'for water retention'. It is likely that an investigator not familiar with the research of Mazzullo *et al.* would regard this as a correct answer. Similarly if the patient was on a schedule which required taking tablets every six hours, and so informed the investigator, this too might be regarded as indicating knowledge of the regimen. As we shall see below it is quite likely that such a patient will be taking three rather than four tablets a day. These problems make the inter-pretation of expert judgement studies a little difficult, as it is not always clear to what extent they are prone to the errors just described. Nevertheless several such studies are summarised in Table 2.2.

It can be seen that the percentage of patients deemed not to have adequate knowledge of dose and schedule varied from 5 to 53, whereas the percentage not having knowledge of the

21

Table 2.2: Patients' understanding of their medication

Investigation	Knowledge criterion used	Per cent judged *not* to have adequate knowledge
Arnhold *et al.* (1970)	Dose	5
Boyd *et al.* (1974)	Amount of dose	9
	Number of doses	14
	Timing of dose	29
	Administration, e.g. with water	5
	Purpose	19
	Name of drug	60
	All of the above	69
Hulka *et al.* (1975b)	Name of drug	40
	Type of insulin	36
Parkin (1976)	Dose and schedule	35
Parkin *et al.* (1976)	Purpose	55
	Name	60
Ellis *et al*, (1979)	Dose and purpose	45
Brody (1980)	Dose and schedule	53
De Wet and Hollingshead (1980)	Purpose	54
Kiernan and Isaacs (1981)	Name	56
	Purpose	41
German *et al.* (1982)	Purpose: patients under age 65	31
	patients over age 65	45
Wartman *et al.* (1983)	Dose and schedule	25
Sanazaro (1985)	Dose and schedule	10

purpose of the drug varied between 19 and 55.

There have been some studies which have attempted to assess patients' understanding of their illnesses. Spelman *et al.* (1966) reported on a series of 80 medical patients and found that, while 85 per cent had a good or reasonable knowledge of their diagnosis, 55 per cent had poor or no understanding of the nature of their illness. Parkin (1976) in a similar study of 134 discharged hospital patients found that 49 per cent had poor or no knowledge of their illness. Ellis, Hopkin, Leitch and Crofton (1979) also assessed patients' knowledge of various aspects of their illness and found that 69 per cent had a poor or no idea of their diagnosis, 88 per cent of the general advice they were given, and 54 per cent of their prognosis. This was despite the fact that the doctors involved thought that they had presented the information 'with great lucidity'.

Another example of expert judgement of patients' understanding is the research of Tuckett, Boulton and Olson (1985). The data base for the investigation consisted of 328 general practice consultations. Judges decided which of the pieces of information provided in the consultation could be considered a 'key point', and the patients were later interviewed to assess their understanding of these key points. In 27 per cent of the consultations where the patient could recall the key points there was a difference in interpretation between the doctor and the patient.

QUASI-BEHAVIOURAL TESTS OF PATIENTS' UNDERSTANDING

In the quasi-behavioural studies patients are asked to specify or demonstrate the behaviours in which they would indulge if given certain instructions. So if the instruction was that the tablets should be taken four times a day, the investigator would ask the patient exactly when the tablets would be taken. The answers to this question have ranged from taking all four tablets in one shot after breakfast to, more commonly, taking four tablets during normal waking hours, and to taking a tablet every six hours throughout the 24 hour clock.

Herman (1973) studied this problem by asking patients who had been prescribed medicines on either a twice, thrice, or four times a day schedule exactly when they would take their tablets. The results are a little hard to summarise as the data are presented in the form of histograms. In the case of tablets to be taken twice daily the inter-dose interval ranged from 3 to 21 hours; in the case of tablets to be taken three times a day, from 0 to 24 hours; and in the case of tablets to be taken four times a day, from 0 to 21 hours. In addition, in 15 per cent of cases patients were unable to specify any schedule at all.

Further evidence that patients are likely to misunderstand timing schedules comes from the study of Alfredsson, Bergman, Eriksson, Gronskog, Norell, Schwartz, and Wiholm (1982). These investigators asked patients who had been instructed to take theophyllines on a three times a day schedule to give details of the times at which they took their medicine. Only 2 per cent reported taking the medicine at eight hour intervals. Intervals between doses ranged from 0 to 18 hours. Similar findings were reported by Norell, Alfredsson, Bergman, Eriksson, Gronskog, Schwarz and Wiholm (1984) in a study of patients' spacing of their doses of three drugs taken on a three times daily basis (hydralazine hydrochloride, slow release potassium chloride, and verapamil hydrochloride). The interval between first and second doses ranged from 3 to 11 hours; between second and third doses from 2 to 10 hours, and the third interval from 8 to 17 hours.

Norell and Granstrom (1980) and Alfredsson and Norell (1981) have used an electronic recording device to assess timing of doses and have confirmed the findings based on patients' reports. In these investigations of patients suffering from glaucoma it was found that only four out of 82 took their pilocarpine at eight hour intervals as prescribed and that the mean lengths of time between first, second and third doses were 6.4, 6.5 and 11.1 hours respectively.

Mazzulo *et al.* (1974) in their study referred to above also collected information of this sort. The instructions and the percentages interpreting them correctly were: 'every six hours', 36 per cent; '30 minutes before meals and at bedtime on an empty stomach', 91 per cent; 'immediately after food four times a day', 85 per cent; 'every four hours as needed for pain', 81 per cent; 'every 12 hours', 63 per cent; and 'take for fluid retention', 42 per cent. Kendrick and Bayne (1982) also asked a similar question. They asked their patients how many tablets they would take in a day if they were told to take a tablet every six hours. Only 22 per cent gave the correct answer.

Watkins, Williams, Martin and Anderson (1967) asked diabetic patients to demonstrate some of the skills needed for them to comply properly with treatment. 52 per cent did not use the correct insulin dosage; 77 per cent did not sterilise their needles properly; 67 per cent made errors in their urine testing; 73 per cent ate their meals on a poor schedule; and 52 per cent did not understand the foot care regimen. Hulka, Kupper, Cassel and Mayo (1975b) asked diabetic patients to demonstrate how to conduct a urine test, but confined their investigation of this topic to those who could recall having been instructed about how to carry out the test. It was found that 97 per cent of this group could conduct the test properly. As the 34 per cent of all of the patients studied by Hulka *et al.* who said that they had not been instructed in how to carry out the test were excluded, this figure is not really directly comparable with the result of Watkins *et al.* More recently Sanazaro (1985) has also assessed diabetics' knowledge of the rules of foot-care and found that 43 per cent did not know them.

Other investigators have studied the kinds of foods that people would avoid given certain dietary instructions. Riley (1966) presented subjects with lists of foods and asked them which they should avoid if told to avoid foods containing starch and sugar. Although only 10 per cent or less failed to realise that the prohibition covered potatoes, bread, and shortcake, 12 per cent would have continued to use sweetened condensed milk; 38 per cent, cream crackers; and the majority were unaware that fruits such as prunes, raisins and chestnuts should be avoided. Another of Riley's questions revealed that people were often unaware of which proprietary medicines contained aspirin. Similar results were reported by Rosenberg (1971) who found that patients with heart disease had little idea of which foods should be avoided if they were on a low sodium diet. The list could of course be extended, but once again it would be expected that the results would be very time and culture bound. However, it is worth recording the probably apocryphal but extremely exemplary tale of the investigation of dietary compliance in diabetics during which the researcher found a diabetic patient tucking into a hearty three-course meal with a monstrously high carbohydrate content. The investigator remarked to the patient that the patient was supposed to be on a diet. The patient's reply was: 'Yes, I know that. I had my diet at 11 o'clock'.

SUMMARY

Investigations of patients' understanding of what they have been told have shown:

(a) Patients often do not know the meanings of the words used by the clinician.

(b) Patients often have their own ideas about illnesses and these often differ from the accepted orthodox ideas. Naturally enough what the clinician says will be interpreted in terms of the patients' own framework of ideas.

25

(c) As measured by the patients' own report, or by expert judgement, or by quasi-behavioural tests, patients often fail to understand what they are told by health care professionals.

(d) Patients are often reluctant to ask for further information even when they would very much like it.

3

Memory for Medical Information

INTRODUCTION

The fact that patients are unable to recall a great deal of what they are told in a consultation is well established. The studies which show this fall into two broad areas. The first of these consists of investigations which have studied recall of the information provided by the doctor in his statements to the patient at the end of the consultation, when the patient is being told what is wrong, what the treatment will be, what the prognosis is, what advice the patient must follow, and what tests and investigations will be necessary. These studies have been reported from a variety of hospital and primary care settings.

The second category of investigations consists of research into patients' recall of informed consent information. In many parts of the world it is now required by law that patients are fully informed of procedures to be carried out on them, and about treatment, both surgical and medical, prescribed for them. It is obviously of interest to know how much of this information is remembered.

In addition to these researches into the recall of information by patients, there have been a number of analogue studies in which healthy volunteers have been required to recall material consisting of sequences of medical statements, which of course do not really apply to them. Interestingly enough the results of these investigations show a remarkable similarity between the success with which real patients recall what they are told and the success with which volunteers recall medical information which is not personally relevant.

There are a number of methodological differences between

27

studies. A very important one is whether the patients are making their first visit with a new illness or not. Obviously if the consultation studied is a repeat visit then the investigator will not know what the patient was told on former occasions, and thus will not be able to assess whether the patient's recall is affected by this.

Another important difference lies in the method used for measuring recall. Sometimes the patient is simply asked to tell the investigator what the doctor has said, a procedure to be referred to as free recall. Sometimes more cues are provided, and the patient is asked what was said in specified areas. So the patient might be asked what was said about the diagnosis, about the proposed treatment, about any investigations, and so on. This will be referred as cued recall. Sometimes the investigator will report using a procedure going even beyond this. Thus some studies have involved persisting with questions until the investigator was sure that the patient cannot recall any more. This will be referred to as probed recall. Finally, sometimes a written set of questions is put to the patient. The questions involved can be either open-ended or multiple-choice. Strictly speaking the multiple choice method is recognition rather than recall.

It would be expected that these procedural differences would affect the amount that patients are reported to remember, and the effects of these differences, as well as the effects of such other variables as the amount of time elapsing between presentation and recall, and the amount of information presented will be discussed further, after the results of the investigations of memory for what the doctor says have been described.

Another problem in assessing recall is the problem of correcting for chance. Suppose that you take a child with a sore throat to a general practitioner. Before the consultation you probably expect that the doctor will prescribe an antibiotic, which, if you had to guess, you would say should be taken four times a day. If it is in term time you also expect to be told to keep the child off school for a couple of days. There is a high probability that these statements will in fact be made by the physician, and so it is likely that any recall score will be inflated by these high base-rate probabilities. Further, many physicians have strong points of view about exercise, weight, smoking and the like. A patient who regularly uses the same doctor will therefore have a high expectation that certain advice about lifestyle change will be given. There are thus a number of ways in which a patient's recall could appear to be higher than it is. This should be more likely to affect results in studies of general practice consultations, where the doctor's views, the illnesses, and the doctor's usual methods of dealing with them are likely to be familiar to the patient. It would also be expected that the effect would be greater the longer the gap between consultation and request for recall. With the passage of time it should become harder to remember on just which occasion often repeated advice was given. Strangely there has been no research into this problem.

THE AMOUNT FORGOTTEN

1. Hospital patients

The earliest investigation was that by Ley and Spelman (1965), who studied 47 medical outpatients' recall of what they were told by the consultant physician they had just seen. The patients had presented with a variety of conditions and, accordingly, had a wide range of statements made to them. Patients were making their first attendance with the illness in question. On average these patients recalled 63 per cent of the information presented to them. The method of assessment was the free recall method, as it was also in the next study.

Ley and Spelman (1967) reported on two further small series of medical outpatients, 22 in each group, who were attending the same clinic as the first series of patients. Once more the patients were making their first visit with their current complaint. In one of these groups of patients average recall was 59 per cent, and in the other it was 61 per cent. These estimates of recall are obviously reasonably consistent with the results of the earlier study.

In 1969 Joyce, Caple, Mason, Reynolds, and Matthews provided data on recall by two sets of patients attending for the first time at a rheumatic diseases clinic. The cued recall method was used. The first group of 30 patients recalled 48 per cent of what they had been told, and the second group consisting of 24 patients recalled 46 per cent. These percentages recalled can be seen to be lower than the percentages recalled by the patients investigated by Ley and Spelman. As will be seen below the main reason for this difference is probably that in the study by

Joyce *et al.* patients were presented with an average of 10 or 12 statements, whereas the patients of Ley and Spelman received only 6 to 8 statements on average.

Kupst, Dresser, Schulman and Paul (1975) using the cued recall method investigated 22 mothers of child patients with congenital heart defects. These were patients in the control group of an experimental study the results of which will be reported subsequently. All patients had been seen on previous occasions, and thus their parent would already know a variety of things about the child's illness. No data were provided on the number of statements made to the mothers, but retention was calculated by subtracting the number of items of information the subject possessed prior to the consultation from the amount known afterwards, and expressing this as a percentage of the amount of new information presented. Thus the amount to be recalled could have been quite small. The average patient recalled 76 per cent of what they had been told when tested immediately after the consultation, and 80 per cent when tested by postal questionnaire one month later.

Another study of rheumatological outpatient first attenders was reported by Anderson, Dodman, Kopelman and Fleming (1979). In the first series 122, and in the second series 29 patients were seen, but as the results for the two series did not differ substantially they were combined into one group. Patients recalled on average 40 per cent of what they had been told. The average patient in this study received twelve statements. The free recall method was used to assess retention.

Reading (1981) studied recall by 36 women inpatients awaiting minor gynaeological surgery. Patients were given ten pieces of information about the procedures. Reading used a method of measuring recall which differed from that used in the studies described above in that he allowed half credit for statements which were half-recalled. This of course means that his results are not strictly comparable with those above. In the event his patients recalled an average of 60 per cent of what they were told, as assessed by the free recall method, and 69 per cent as assessed by probed recall.

The results of all these investigations are summarised in Table 3.1, which also provides details of time elapsing between presentation and recall of the information.

Table 3.1: Recall of information by hospital patients

Investigation	Patients	Mean number of statements made	Delay before recall	Mean % recalled	Method of assessing recall
Ley and Spelman (1965)	47 new medical outpatients	5.6	0–80 minutes	63	Free
Ley and Spelman (1967)	(a) 22 new medical outpatients	7.0	0–80 minutes	61	Free
	(b) 22 new medical outpatients	7.9	0–80 minutes	59	Free
Joyce et al (1969)	(a) 30 new rheumatological outpatients	9.5	Nil	48	Cued
	(b) 24 new rheumatological outpatients	11.9	1–4 weeks	46	Cued
Kupst et al. (1975)	22 repeat visit cardiac patients	?	Nil / 1 month	76 / 80	Cued / Written
Anderson et al. (1979)	151 new rheumatological outpatients	12.1	Nil	40	Free
Reading (1981)	(a) 20 gynaecological inpatients	10.0	Nil	70 / 80	Free / Probed
	(b) 16 gynaecological inpatients	10.0	3h	47 / 55	Free / Probed

2. General practice patients

Ley, Bradshaw, Eaves, and Walker (1973) assessed the recall of 20 general practice new attenders. These patients recalled an average of 50 per cent of the seven or so statements made to them. The free recall method was used in this study.

A similar degree of recall, 56 per cent, was shown by a larger series of 157 patients seen by Ley *et al.* (1976b). Once again patients were first attenders. The average number of statements made to them was seven, and recall was assessed by a written open-ended questionnaire.

Hulka, Cassel, Kupper and Burdette (1976), Hulka, Kupper, Cassel and Rabineau (1975c), and Hulka (1979) studied the success with which information was transmitted from physician to patient in samples of patients suffering from diabetes, in pregnant women, and in mothers of young children. A large proportion of these patients were seen in a family practice setting, and many were not first attenders. Hulka *et al.* use a communication score, which is the proportion of items of information that the doctor wishes the patient to know which are in fact known to the patient. In the sample of 242 diabetics this score showed that patients recalled on average 67 per cent of what their doctor had told them, or perhaps more accurately, what their doctor wished them to know. In the case of mothers of infants the modal percentage recalled was approximately 88 per cent, and in the case of pregnant women 68 per cent. (The figures are approximate because they have been read from graphs.) These investigations involved 523 infants, and 363 pregnant women. Retention was assessed by the cued recall method.

An investigation of a sample of 50 patients seen in a family practice clinic was reported by Bertakis (1977). This investigator found that patients recalled on average 62 per cent of what they had been told. The average number of items of information presented to each patient was thirteen. This study therefore reports a relatively high level of recall. The patients involved were once more first attenders, and cued recall was used.

Tuckett, Boulton and Olson (1985) also report a high level of recall. These investigators studied 328 patients seen by 16 general practitioners. Patients in this investigation were probably not first attenders, nor were the results reported in a fashion which allows direct comparison with those reported

Table 3.2: Recall of information by general practice patients

Investigation	Patients	Mean number of statements made	Delay before recall	Mean % recalled	Method of assessing recall
Ley et al. (1973)	20 new patients	7.2	< 5 min	50	Free
Ley et al. (1976b)	157 new patients	5.1	1 to 2 weeks	56	Cued, written
Hulka et al. (1975c)	242 diabetics (repeats)	?	?	67	Cued
Hulka, Cassel et al. (1975)	(a) 363 pregnant women	?	?	68	Cued
	(b) 523 infants	?	?	88	Cued
Bertakis (1977)	50 new patients	13.4	Nil	62	Cued
Tuckett et al. (1985)	328 probably includes repeats	?	?	(only 10 failed to recall all key points)	Probed

above. However Tuckett *et al.* found that only ten per cent of their patients failed to remember all the 'key points' that they were told. Possible reasons for the apparent discrepancy between this result and that of the other studies will be discussed below. Tuckett *et al.* do not provide data on the number of statements with which their patients were presented. Retention was assessed by probed recall.

Table 3.2 summarises these studies.

3. Studies of informed consent materials

Unfortunately the descriptions of the informed consent studies to be considered often fail to provide much detail. This makes for some difficulty in their interpretation as investigations of patients' recall. It will be remembered that the information to be recalled has been given to the patients for legal or other reasons. There has been a great deal of interest in how well such information has been remembered.

Leeb, Bowers and Lynch (1976) reported on recall of such information by 100 patients undergoing plastic reconstructive surgery. In this study patients were not all given the same amount of information. Despite this the recall measure was the number of statements recalled, expressed as a percentage of 10, seven days after presentation. Obviously this unusual manoeuvre on the part of the investigators makes for some difficulty in the interpretation of the results. A further feature of this investigation was that patients were told that recall would be requested at a later date. In the event patients recalled 32 per cent as measured by the scoring procedure. Note, however, that as many patients received more than ten statements this figure is an overestimate. It is probable that this study used free recall. The information was presented orally.

Morrow, Gootnick and Schmale (1978) investigated recall by 77 cancer patients. Thirty-seven were tested for immediate recall of what they had read in an informed consent statement, and the others, whose results will be described later, were tested after they had been allowed to keep this written information at home for a few days. Cued recall was used and patients recalled from 35 to 95 per cent of what they had read of the various categories of information presented, with a median recall of 88 per cent.

Cheadle and Morgan (1975) investigated psychiatric patients' recall of what was said to them at a clinical review interview. Cued recall yielded a mean recall of 41 per cent immediately after the interview, and of 31 per cent when the patients were interviewed one week later.

Twenty cardiac patients were studied by Robinson and Merav (1976). These patients were seen before operation when the information was presented, and then 4 to 6 months afterwards, when recall was requested. Two measures of recall were used. The first was cued recall and the second was probed recall. Cued recall yielded a mean percentage recall of 29 per cent, and probed recall of 42 per cent.

Kennedy and Lillehaugen (1979) found that 50 per cent of 40 patients with cancer could recall giving consent to the use of research drugs, and 60 per cent could recall giving consent to research tests five to seven days after giving such consent.

In a study of recall by patients with breast cancer by Muss, White, Michielutte, Richards, Cooper, Williams, Stuart and Spurr (1979) 100 patients were interviewed 0 to 24 months after the commencement of chemotherapy. The information presented had been in written form supplemented by the opportunity to ask questions. Recall was assessed by a questionnaire, either administered orally by the researcher or in written form. Patients' mean knowledge of the drugs they were taking was 34 per cent, of possible side-effects 69 per cent, and of the purpose of treatment, 47 per cent. Once more the design of the study makes interpretation difficult. Thus for example some of the patients who had been taking the drugs before being asked to answer the questions had experienced or were experiencing some of the side-effects.

Priluck, Robertson and Buettner (1979) investigated recall by 100 patients who had undergone surgery for detached retina. Cued recall was used and patients recalled on average 57 per cent of what they had been told. The information was presented orally.

A multiple choice test was used by Bergler, Pennington, Metcalfe and Freis (1980) to assess how much patients remembered of the informed consent presented to them. The average amount remembered was 72 per cent when these 39 hypertensive patients were tested two hours after being presented with the information. The information had been conveyed to patients in an informed consent document, supplemented by the opportunity to ask questions.

A written test of memory was also used in a study of 200 patients with cancer by Cassileth, Zupkis, Sutton-Smith and March (1980). This time the questions were open-ended. On average these patients recalled 69 per cent of what they had been told in a written form, backed up by oral supplementation.

Jaffe (1981) reported on recall of information about tardive dyskinesia, a possible side-effect of some neuroleptic drugs, by relatives of psychiatric patients for whom it was proposed to prescribe such medication. Mean percentage recall five to ten weeks later was 33 per cent.

Recall of informed consent materials was also investigated by Taub and Baker (1983). Subjects were volunteers who were to participate in studies of basic visual processes in the elderly. The informed consent materials were read by the subjects who were then asked questions to see whether they had understood what they had read, and were given appropriate feedback if they had not. Recall of the materials was tested two to three weeks later, and it was found that the mean recall was 38 per cent.

These results are summarised in Table 3.3.

4. Analogue studies

In the analogue studies to be described healthy volunteers are given a set of medical statements to remember. The sets of statements used are collections of statements which could well be made to a real patient, but in the analogue investigations they are not true of the person receiving them. The main advantage of analogue investigations is the degree of experimental control they permit. Their main disadvantage is of course that because of the differences between the analogue and the real-life situations, findings derived from them will not necessarily apply in the real situation. As it transpires analogue studies have yielded results very similar to those obtained in the clinic.

Ley and Spelman (1967) randomly assigned 162 volunteer subjects to receiving either six, nine or twelve medical statements. Memory was assessed by the free recall method and the three groups recalled respectively, 64, 53 and 41 per cent.

In a study by Ley (1972b) 82 subjects were randomly assigned to receiving six or twelve statements. As assessed by the free recall method those receiving six statements remembered 64 per cent, and those receiving twelve statements

Table 3.3: Patients' recall of informed consent information

Investigation	Patients	Mean number of statements made	Delay before recall	Mean % recalled	Method of assessing recall
Leeb et al. (1976)	100 plastic surgery	?	Within 7 days	32	? Free
Cheadle and Morgan (1975)	113 psychiatric	?	Nil 1 week	41 31	Cued Cued
Robinson and Merav (1976)	20 cardiac	?	4 to 6 months	29 42	Free Probed
Morrow et al. (1978)	37 cancer	?	Nil	35–95	Cued
Muss et al. (1979)	100 breast cancer	?	0 to 24 months	34–69	Cued, written
Kennedy and Lillehaugen (1979)	40 cancer	?	5–7 days	55	Cued, written
Priluck et al. (1979)	100 detached retina	?	4 days	57	Cued
Bergler et al. (1980)	39 hypertensives	?	2 hours 3 months	72 61	Cued, written
Cassileth et al. (1980)	200 cancer	?	< 1 day	69	Cued, written
Jaffe (1981)	19 relatives	?	5–10 weeks	33	Cued, written
Taub and Baker (1983)	100 elderly	?	2–3 weeks	38	Cued, written

recalled 52 per cent.

Ley (1979a) reported on free recall by 63 volunteers and 42 nurses given fifteen statements. The lay volunteers recalled 33 per cent, but the nurses recalled 63 per cent. This difference, it will be argued later, was due to the material being more meaningful to the nurses because of their greater medical knowledge. In the same paper it was reported that 12 volunteers given eight statements to recall had recalled 34 per cent, 18 given ten statements had recalled 34 per cent, and 12 given sixteen statements had recalled 28 per cent.

5. More limited information

A number of investigations have studied patients' recall of more limited aspects of the information presented to them. Thus Hulka, Kupper, Cassel, Efird and Burdette (1975a) reported on patients' scheduling misconceptions, i.e. the proportion of drugs for which the patient does not recall the right dose and/or frequency of use. The samples of patients studied included 123 with congestive cardiac failure and 234 with diabetes. For both groups the proportion of such errors was 0.17, suggesting a fairly high level of recall of this sort of information, but many of these patients had had multiple consultations about their illnesses, which in some cases were of some years' duration.

Bain (1977), in a sample of 480 general practice consultations, found that 63 per cent of patients could recall the name of their medication, 77 per cent could recall the frequency with which it should be taken, and 75 per cent could recall the length of time for which they should continue to take the medicine. Patients were tested for recall within an hour of the consultation.

Further information about patients' recall of their treatment regimen comes from an investigation by Crichton, Smith and Demanuele (1978), who found that free recall of information presented by the pharmacist was 78 per cent after one day's delay, and 70 per cent at seven days. Additional evidence of forgetting was found by Brody (1980), who, using cued recall, found that 53 per cent of patients made at least one mistake in recalling their treatment regimen. Bartlett, Grayson, Barker, Levine, Golden and Libber (1984) also provided data on patients' recall of treatment advice. Patients were not first attenders and most were suffering from a chronic illness. Recall was assessed 1–2 weeks after the consultation. Mean recall was 86 per cent. Note, however, that in this study (and in the samples of Hulka *et al.* and Crichton *et al.*), all or many of the patients should have been taking the medicines for some days or weeks, and thus been frequently exposed to a container labelled with the name of the medicine and instructions for its use. This contrasts with the investigations of Bain and Brody, where the patient was asked to recall immediately after seeing the physician.

In a study of obese patients' recall of dietary advice Bradshaw, Ley, Kincey and Bradshaw (1975) found that their obese clients could recall 34 per cent of the instructions they had been given. These investigators also reported on two analogue studies of memory for dietary advice. In one of these subjects recalled 28 per cent of the advice, and in the other 34 per cent.

In another analogue study Ley, Goldman, Bradshaw, Kincey and Walker (1972) investigated recall of leaflets informing patients of X-ray examination procedures and telling them how to prepare for these tests. It was found that subjects recalled 75 per cent of the contents of a barium meal leaflet, and 69 per cent of the information in a cholecystogram leaflet.

Thus these clinical and analogue studies provide further evidence of forgetting.

METHODOLOGICAL PROBLEMS

As was mentioned in the introduction to this chapter the investigations reported have differed in a number of procedural ways which might be expected to affect results. It will be worthwhile examining some of these before looking at some of the correlates of how much is remembered.

Not all studies have used as their subjects patients attending for the first time with a new illness. This was true of the investigations of Kupst *et al.* (1975), Hulka, Cassel *et al.* (1975), Hulka *et al.* (1975c), Muss *et al.* (1979), and probably of Tuckett *et al.* (1985). Mean percentages recalled in these studies tended to be higher than those in studies which investigated recall of information new to the patient. The median of the mean percentages recalled for researches involving second or later visits was 68 per cent, whereas for first visits it was 53 per cent. In addition Tuckett *et al.* reported that only 10 per cent of their 328 patients failed to recall the information given to them. This contrasts sharply with the findings of Ley and Spelman (1965, 1967), who found that only 22 per cent of their 91 patients recalled everything, Joyce *et al.* (1969), none of whose 54 patients recalled everything, and Robinson and Merav (1976), none of whose 20 patients recalled everything. It also contrasts with the finding of Ley and Spelman (1967) that only 12 out of 162 subjects (7 per cent) in their analogue experiment recalled everything.

While this evidence would make it appear that patients making a repeat visit recall more, interpretation is not straightforward as these investigations differ in other ways as well. For example the number of statements made to patients varies as does the method of assessing recall. Fortunately one investigation provides evidence from within its sample of patients that patients who have been ill longer, and thus presumably have made more visits, are more likely to be able to recall what their physician wants them to know. Hulka *et al.* (1975c) reported that the percentages of patients who had been ill for less than a year, 1 to 3 years, and more than 3 years, who could remember more than 50 per cent were 63, 68, and 83 per cent respectively.

A second major methodological variable likely to affect amount recalled is the method by which recall is elicited. It would be expected that the more cueing and the more probing the greater will be the recall. Any simple test of this possibility by comparing rates of recall in studies which used cueing and probing with rates in those studies which did not is confounded by other differences between studies. Fortunately two investigations have reported within-study comparisons of free and probed recall. Unfortunately the design of both was such that the same subjects were used to assess both free and probed recall. In both studies subjects were first asked to recall freely what they had been told and then were exposed to cues and probes.

In the first of these Robinson and Merav (1976) found that mean percentage recall increased from 29 per cent in the free condition to 42 per cent in the probed condition. These findings are echoed by Reading (1981) who found mean recall in the free condition to be 60 per cent and in the probed condition 69 per cent. Whether these increases are due to the cueing and probing or just due to a second attempt at recall cannot be ascertained as appropriate controls are missing. However, it would be prudent to be cautious when comparing the results of investigations using cueing with those using free recall. At least a prima facie case has been made out for supposing that cueing will lead to higher estimates of recall, and, of course, such an expectation is consistent with what is known of the psychology of memory in general.

A third methodological difference between studies is the length of time elapsing between presentation and recall. It would be expected that the longer the delay the poorer would be the recall. The evidence in favour of this hypothesis is rather weak in investigations of recall of medical information. Several studies have provided data on this relationship within their samples. Ley and Spelman (1965, 1967) found that in none of their three samples of outpatients was there a significant relationship between time elapsing and recall. The time range involved was 10–80 minutes. Joyce et al. (1969) found that patients tested immediately after the consultation recalled 48 per cent, whereas those tested after a delay of one to four weeks recalled 46 per cent. A further negative result comes from the study by Muss et al. (1980) who found no correlation between delay and recall over a period of 0 to 24 months. This result must, however, be treated with some caution, as it is likely that patients might well have received multiple exposures to the information if they had experienced a longer delay, and, as part of the information to be recalled concerned side-effects, would be more likely to have experienced these, and thus be more aware of them. Ley (1972b) in an analogue investigation also found no relation between recall and delay. Subjects tested immediately recalled 58 per cent, while those tested after 20 minutes recalled 56 per cent. Crichton et al. (1978) found that patients' recall of medication-related information was 78 per cent after one day, and 70 per cent after one week. Jaffe (1981) reported that mean recall of information, in the subset of relatives whose recall was assessed on two occasions, was 29 per cent five to ten weeks after the consultation, but 43 per cent at four to six months. Finally in this catalogue of negative results, Phillips and Little (1980) found no correlation between mothers' recall of advice about preventing accidental poisoning of children and time elapsing since the information was presented.

41

Two investigations which did not report whether the results were statistically significant reported poorer recall after delay. In the first of these Cheadle and Morgan (1975) reported that immediate recall was 41 per cent, and recall after one week was 31 per cent. Bergler *et al.* (1980) found recall after two hours to be 72 per cent, and after three months to be 62 per cent. A third study, Reading (1981) reported mean immediate free recall to be 70 per cent and three hour recall to be 47 per cent. For probed recall the percentages recalled were 80 and 55 respectively. The results were significant. Unfortunately Reading used four interviewers who differed significantly in the amount of recall they elicited, and those obtaining the highest recall scores conducted 75 per cent of the immediate interviews but only 38 per cent of the delayed interviews. This could have affected the results.

Thus overall there is only very weak evidence of an association between delay and recall. The majority of studies fail to find any significant relationship, two which might have found such an association do not report whether their results are significant, and the one which does report a significant association confounded possible interviewer effects with the effects of delay. This failure to find an effect of delay is surprising in the light of the literature on the experimental psychology of memory, which would clearly lead to the expectation of such an effect.

Having briefly discussed these potentially confounding variables it is now time to consider some more clinically important ones. These include the relation between amount recalled and (a) amount presented, (b) patient characteristics such as age, intelligence, education, medical knowledge, and anxiety level, and (c) the nature of the material presented. In this last category will be discussed not only the content of the material but also recall of material in relation to its serial position.

THE RELATIONSHIP BETWEEN AMOUNT PRESENTED AND RECALL

In the analogue studies by Ley and Spelman (1967), and Ley (1979a) a clear relationship between amount presented and percentage recalled can be seen. These analogue studies provide data on reasonably large samples of volunteers given six, nine, twelve or fifteen statements to recall. The 70 subjects who received six statements recalled 64 per cent; the 54 who were given nine statements recalled 53 per cent; the 70 who were given twelve statements recalled 44 per cent; and the 63 who were given fifteen statements recalled 33 per cent.

Some of the clinical studies also report a relationship between amount presented and recall. Ley and Spelman (1965), Anderson *et al.* (1979), and Ley (1979a) reported that the more statements made to a patient the greater the percentage forgotten, and Joyce *et al.* (1979) just missed finding this relationship (p <0.10). These hospital outpatient studies are therefore consistent in finding that the more information presented the greater will be the proportion forgotten. Note that it is the *proportion* forgotten that increases, and that this is quite compatible with patients given more information knowing more about their condition than those given less. The finding is therefore not an argument for providing patients with less information.

Confidence in the finding of greater proportional forgetting with increasing amounts presented is increased by the striking similarity between the analogue and hospital investigations. Figure 3.1 shows the lines of best fit between amount presented and mean percentage recalled for both the analogue and the hospital data. It can be seen that these lines of best fit are almost identical for the two sets of studies.

For whatever reasons the picture is not so clear in the case of the general practice investigations. The patients of Ley *et al.* (1973) received on average 7.2 statements and recalled an average of 50 per cent, whereas those of Ley *et al.* (1976b) recalled an average of 56 per cent of the mean 5.1 statements made to them. Using the hospital regression equation to predict recall these percentages would have been expected to be 61 and 67 respectively, which as the predictions are of mean recall is not very accurate. In the case of the study by Bertakis (1977) the prediction is even further out. Patients in that study recalled on average 62 per cent of 13.4 statements presented to them, against a predicted 42 per cent. Why these general practice data should behave so differently from the hospital data is quite unclear, and further research is needed to shed light on this problem. However, it is tempting to wonder whether the greater predictability (postulated above) of what the general practitioner is going to say might have contributed to these differences between general practice and hospital studies.

Figure 3.1: Relationship between number of statements presented and the percentage recalled in analogue samples (solid circles) and clinic samples (open circles). Also shown are the lines of best fit. The upper is for the clinic samples and the lower for the analogue samples.

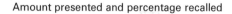

Amount presented and percentage recalled

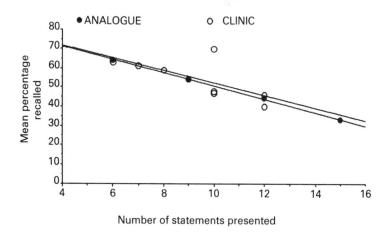

Number of statements presented

PATIENTS' CHARACTERISTICS AND FORGETTING

The relationship between age and recall has been investigated in several studies with mixed results. In both clinical and analogue studies the commonest finding has been that there is no significant relationship between the age of the patient or subject and the amount recalled. Thus Joyce *et al.* (1969), Anderson *et al.* (1979), Cassileth *et al.* (1980), and Ley and Spelman (1967), for two of their analogue samples, all report no significant relationship between age and recall.

However, Ley and Spelman (1965) reported a positive relationship between age and recall, the older patients remembering more, whereas Ley *et al.* (1976b) found that patients over the age of 65 recalled less of what they were told. Finally, for one of their analogue samples Ley and Spelman (1967) reported a significant negative relationship between age and recall. It is probably prudent to conclude that age within the young adult and middle-age range does not affect recall, but that it is possible that the elderly might have more difficulty in remembering.

From the clinical study by Ley and Spelman (1965) and the analogue studies of Ley and Spelman (1967) it would appear that the correlation between intellectual level and recall is of the order of +0.20. Although none of the correlations in these four samples was significant when taken individually, all were of the same magnitude. A relationship of this size is probably of little clinical interest, so for all practical purposes intelligence will not be a major factor in determining recall. Similarly in the studies of Bertakis (1977), and of Kupst *et al.* (1975) educational level has a low but statistically significant relationship to recall, but once more it is probably of little clinical significance.

Analogue studies have revealed a consistent relationship between the subject's overall level of medical knowledge and recall. Ley and Spelman (1967) reported correlations of +0.33, +0.52 and +0.35 for their samples who received six, nine or twelve statements to recall. It is also tempting to interpret the finding of vastly superior recall by nurses (reported above), to their greater medical knowledge.

The patient's level of anxiety has been found to be related to recall in four studies. Ley and Spelman (1965) reported a Yerkes–Dodson 'inverted U' relationship between patient anxiety and recall, the patients with moderate anxiety recalling more than those with higher or lower anxiety. However, this finding has not been confirmed by Anderson *et al.* (1979) who found a simple positive linear relationship between these variables. A positive correlation between anxiety and recall has also been reported by Kupst *et al.* (1975) and Leeb *et al.* (1976). All four studies agree on the finding that low anxiety is associated with poorer recall, and three of them agree that high anxiety is associated with superior recall.

The findings of these investigations of the relationship between patients' characteristics and recall are summarised in Table 3.4. In the table a 'p' value has been recorded for studies which did not provide a correlation coefficient or sufficient details for one to be calculated from the data provided.

CONTENT AND OTHER FACTORS AND RECALL

In the early study by Ley and Spelman (1985) it was reported that patients best recalled statements about diagnosis, and recalled worst statements giving them instructions and advice.

45

Table 3.4: Relationships between patients' characteristics and recall

Investigation	Age	Intelligence	Education	Anxiety	Medical knowledge
(a) Clinical studies					
Ley and Spelman (1965)	+ 0.38*	+ 0.24	—	< 0.05	—
Joyce et al. (1969)	n.s.	—	—	—	—
Bertakis (1977)	—	—	< 0.05	—	—
Kupst et al. (1975)	—	—	—	+ 0.18	—
Leeb et al. (1976)	—	—	< 0.05	< 0.05	—
Ley et al. (1976)	< 0.05	—	—	—	—
Anderson et al. (1979)	n.s.	—	—	< 0.05	—
Cassileth et al. (1980)	n.s.	—	—	—	—
(b) Analogue studies					
Ley and Spelman (1967) Group given:					
6 statements	− 0.16	+ 0.18	—	—	+ 0.33*
9 statements	− 0.30*	+ 0.19	—	—	+ 0.52*
12 statements	− 0.09	+ 0.26	—	—	+ 0.35*

Notes: * $p < 0.05$; n.s. = not significant; $< 0.05 = p < 0.05$.

Of diagnostic statements 86 per cent were recalled as opposed to 44 per cent of advice and instruction statements and 62 per cent of other statements. This finding is far from universal. A similar, but non-significant, pattern was reported by Ley *et al.* (1973); whereas Ley *et al.* (1976b) found that diagnostic statements were better recalled than instructions, but not better than other statements. Further Anderson *et al.* (1979) found no differences in recall between these categories of statement.

This confusion of results is perhaps explicable as Ley (1972b) has shown that the better recall of diagnostic statements, when it occurs, is to a large extent explained by two more basic phenomena. The first of these is that in the case of recall of medical, as well as most other statements, there is a strong primacy effect. People recall better what they are told first. Secondly, people recall better what they consider most important. In situations where the patient is told about the diagnosis first, (a not uncommon situation), and/or where the patient considers the diagnosis to be the most important piece of information, then it would be expected that the diagnosis would be better recalled. Where these conditions do not obtain then there will be less tendency for better recall of diagnosis.

Evidence concerning a primacy effect, i.e. that people remember best what they are told first, in relation to memory for medical information, comes from three analogue studies. Ley and Spelman (1967) found that their subjects recalled 56 per cent of the first third of the material with which they were presented, as compared with 45 per cent and 42 per cent of the subsequent thirds. Ley (1972b) reported memory for the first half of information presented to be 62 per cent, and for the second half 53 per cent. Subjects in the first of these investigations received six, nine, or twelve statements to recall, and those in the second six or twelve. When the number of statements is considerably greater than this, the primacy effect, at least in relation to large proportions, e.g. thirds or halves, of the material, seems to disappear. Thus, Ley (1982a) found that recall of quite a large amount of information about glaucoma and its treatment showed a primacy effect only on the first few statements. Mean recall of successive thirds was 41, 38, and 44 per cent.

In analogue studies the perceived importance of a medical statement is correlated with the probability that it will be recalled. Ley and Spelman (1967) had subjects rate and rank how important a statement would be to patients if it were true of them. There was consistency amongst ratings and rankings and the results showed that diagnostic statements were considered the most important, and instructions and advice the least important. For example, in the ranking task, in 65 per cent of rankings a diagnostic statement was ranked as most important, but instruction/advice statements were only ranked as most important on 16 per cent of occasions. Further the rated importance of a statement was a good predictor of whether it would be recalled (Ley, 1972b). A further investigation also reported by Ley (1972b) found that recall of the more important half presented was 64 per cent whereas only 51 per cent of the half judged less important was recalled.

These results are summarised in Table 3.5.

SUMMARY

The findings reviewed above can be summarised as follows.

(a) Patients often forget a great deal of what they are told. Because the degree of forgetting recorded in a study depends on a variety of factors such as how much material was presented, how recall was elicited, and so on, it is impossible to put an absolute figure on the amount forgotten.

(b) Perhaps surprisingly, the time elapsing between presentation and recall of the material is very little, if at all, related to how much is recalled. This suggests that patients retain well what they can recall immediately after the consultation.

(c) The number of statements presented in both the hospital and analogue studies is linearly related to mean percentage recalled. Further the regression equations describing this relationship are strikingly similar for the two groups of studies. In the studies of general practice patients this relationship, however, is not apparent. There is no obvious reason for this discrepancy.

(d) In general there appears to be no consistent relationship between the age of the patient and the amount recalled. There is, however, some suggestion that patients over age 65 perhaps have poorer recall.

Table 3.5: The relationship between primacy, rated importance and recall

Investigation	Material	Percentage recalled			p
(a) Primacy					
Ley and Spelman (1967)	First third presented	56			
	Second third presented	45			
	Last third presented	42			< 0.001
Ley (1972b)	First half presented	62			
	Second half presented	53			< 0.01
Ley (1982a)	First third presented	41			
	Second third presented	38			
	Last third presented	44			n.s.
(b) Rated importance					
Ley (1972b)	More important half	64			
	Less important half	51			< 0.01
		SampleA*	B*	C*	
Ley (1972b)	Most important third	79	59	51	A < 0.10
	Next in importance	64	57	46	B < 0.01
	Least important third	55	40	25	C < 0.01

Note: A*, B*, C*, = samples given six, nine or twelve statements to recall.

(e) The patient's intellectual and educational level have a low but relatively consistent relationship to recall.

(f) The individual's general level of medical knowledge has also, in analogue studies, shown a consistent relationship to recall.

(g) Patients with low anxiety recall less than those with higher levels of anxiety, and the balance of the evidence suggests that patients with a high level of anxiety recall best of all.

(h) There appears to be a primacy effect in recall of medical information. People recall best what they are told first.

(i) The perceived importance of a statement is related to the probability of its being recalled. If people regard a medical statement as important then they will remember it better than if it is not regarded as important.

Amongst these findings there are few surprises. Perhaps the most surprising is the lack of relationship between time elapsing since presentation and recall. A number of possible explanations of this finding can be suggested. First, consider the situation of a patient who has been to a general practitioner or hospital to find out what is wrong. On return to family or friends that patient is likely to be asked for details of the consultation, the diagnosis, the treatment and so on. This rehearsal of the information is likely to fix the details in memory more firmly, especially as they might well have to be repeated to a number of inquirers, either by the patient, or by those already familiar with them in the patient's hearing.

In addition, in so far as some of the information might be concerned with treatment or the side-effects thereof, if the request to recall is sufficiently delayed there will possibly have been repetition of some of this information by pharmacists, or in writing on the medication. Further, with the passage of time, the patient might well have experienced some of the side-effects. All these factors would be expected to increase measured recall.

The relative lack of a drop in recall with the passage of time might also be due to the fact that the material in question is highly personally relevant, and that which survives the period immediately after the consultation is, as we have seen, likely to be judged as important by the patient.

The failure to find a consistent tendency for older people to recall less is interesting in view of studies of subjective reports of forgetting of compliance-related information. Thus Klein *et al.* (1984) reported that the percentage of their subjects who claimed that they failed to take their medication properly because of forgetfulness was 27 per cent in those under age 65, and 21 per cent in those over 65. These authors also reported the results of a community survey in which it was found that the percentage of hypertensive patients under age 65 attributing their non-compliance to lapses of memory was 14 per cent, whereas in those over 65 it was 13 per cent. Further evidence on this topic has been provided by Martin (1986), who found that an older sample reported themselves to be significantly less likely to forget to take their medicines, and to forget appointments than did a sample of younger people. The cynical view that these findings arose because the older samples were more likely to forget the number of times they had forgotten is hard to hold in the light of further findings in these studies. First, in Martin's investigation the older sample did not consistently report fewer memory difficulties than the younger sample. For example they reported greater difficulties in remembering names and telephone numbers than the younger sample. Secondly, in the Klein *et al.* study younger and older patients did not differ in compliance, and in Martin's research the older sample did in fact miss fewer appointments than the younger sample as judged by an objective record of a subset of the appointments they were supposed to keep. Thus the self-report data are consistent with the available objective data.

The relationship between overall level of medical knowledge and recall is presumably a reflection of the more general finding that meaningful material is better recalled than less meaningful material. In the present case higher medical knowledge would be expected to increase recall in one of two ways. First, it is likely that the more medical knowledge one has the more likely it is that one will already have knowledge of the condition and its implications. Thus remembering the diagnosis might be all that is necessary to recall the treatment, investigations, and other features of a condition. Secondly, even if knowledge does not extend to the condition in question, because of the higher degree of familiarity with medical terminology it is likely that the information will be easier to process and thus recall.

The primacy effect seems to be a relatively consistent finding in studies of memory for meaningful continuous prose. Thus

Ley and Spelman (1967) reported on early studies by Jersild (1929) and Doob (1953), as well as their own studies which found that there was a strong tendency for the material presented first to be better recalled. From the investigations of Jersild (1929) and Ley (1982a) it would appear that even if large amounts of material are presented, the effect is still found in that the first one to three statements made are better recalled. For example, in the study of memory for information about glaucoma and its treatment briefly reported by Ley (1982a), 78 per cent of subjects recalled the first statement they read and 69 per cent the second, compared with average recall over all statements of 41 per cent.

To summarise, the problem of patients' forgetting is a major one. The patient who is likely to forget most is the patient with a low level of medical knowledge, a low level of anxiety, lower intelligence, and poorer education. Unless the patient is over 65 years old age will probably not be an important factor. Patients will remember best what they are told first, and what they consider most important.

Some methods for improving recall and their effectiveness will be considered in later chapters.

4

The Problem of Patients' Non-compliance

INTRODUCTION

The problem of the extent to which patients follow the advice given to them by health care professionals is a major one. As we shall see patients often fail to follow advice. Further this non-compliance, leading as it often does to extra visits to the doctor, unnecessary hospitalisation and so on, can be extremely costly, not only to the individual involved, but also to the health care system as a whole.

Interest in the problem of non-compliance has a lengthy history. Indeed Hippocrates in c.200 BC, in his work 'Decorum', mentioned the problem, advising the physician to be alert to the faults of patients which make them lie about their taking of the medicines prescribed, and, when things go wrong, refusing to confess that they have not been taking their medicine (Jones 1967). However, interest in the problem as reflected in publications in the scientific literature, rose from 25 publications in the 1950s, to 168 in the 1960s, to 810 in the 1970s, to 744 in the period 1980–1984 (Koltun and Stone, 1986). Indeed there are now journals which devote a great deal of their space to this problem, e.g. *Patient Education and Counselling*, and one which is entirely devoted to it, *The Journal of Compliance in Health Care*.

Nor have the ethical problems involved in the concept of compliance and in its manipulation been ignored (Jonsen 1979). Indeed the use of the term 'non-compliance' has itself been criticised, because it smacks of authoritarian relationships, and tends to perpetuate the unequal relationship between doctors and other health professionals and patients (Stimson,

1974; Tuckett *et al.*, 1986). For present purposes these problems will not be discussed in detail, but it is clear that the minimal ethical requirements for attempts to influence compliance are that the patient should be fully and accurately informed of both the risks and benefits of the advocated treatment and of the main alternative treatments, and that there should be regular review to ensure that the patient has the opportunity to indicate a change of mind.

THE MEASUREMENT OF COMPLIANCE

Areas in which compliance has been studied cover almost all areas of advice from clinicians to patients. These have ranged from compliance with short-term antibiotic regimens to compliance with advice about major lifestyle changes designed to reduce obesity or lessen the chances of developing heart disease. The majority of studies have been concerned with compliance with medication regimens where non-compliance has been defined as exhibiting one or more of the following behaviours:

(a) not taking enough medicine;
(b) taking too much medicine;
(c) not observing the correct interval between doses;
(d) not observing the correct duration of treatment;
(e) taking additional non-prescribed medications.

There have also been different definitions of what is deemed adequate compliance in terms of the amount of non-compliance allowed before a patient is labelled non-compliant. Thus the percentage of medicine the patient needs to take to be judged compliant has usually been in the range 75–100 per cent, although it has sometimes been lower.

Methods for assessing the extent to which patients are following advice properly have included:

(a) patients' reports;
(b) pill and bottle counts;
(c) blood and urine tests;
(d) mechanical devices;
(e) direct observation;

54

(f) outcome – the progress of the illness or condition;

(g) clinician's judgement.

Because of the ease with which they can be obtained the use of patients' reports of their adherence to the prescribed regimen has been the most popular method. There are obvious potential problems with this method. First, patients might intentionally deceive the examiner. Secondly, patients might forget instances of non-compliance and thus under-report these. Thirdly, patients might think they are complying and so report, but in fact, because of lack of understanding of the regimen, not realise the extent of their non-compliance. It is clearly wise to try to reduce patients' motivation to deceive the examiner by making the interviewer's approach non-judgemental and by indicating that non-compliance is a not uncommon pheno- menon. For example, Haynes, Taylor, Sackett, Gibson, Bernholz and Muckherjee (1980b) introduced their compliance questions by saying — 'People often have difficulty taking their pills for one reason or another and we are interested in finding out any problems that occur so that we can understand them better'. The second problem can, in theory, be reduced by asking patients to keep some form of written record. The main problems with this are that this method is also subject to faking, and it imposes a further compliance task on the patient. The third problem can be overcome by ensuring that the questions asked provide the examiner with enough data to to form a clear picture of the patient's compliance. For example, just how much medicine was taken, at what times, and in what relationship to meals.

Perhaps the most sophisticated interview approach to date has been that of Morisky, Green and Levine (1986) who devised a set of questions which demonstrated their validity in predicting blood pressure control over a five year period. The authors also provide information on the reliability of the ques- tions. The questions are:

(a) Do you ever forget to take your medicine?

(b) Are you careless at times about taking your medicine?

(c) When you feel better do you sometimes stop taking your medicine?

(d) Sometimes when you feel worse do you sometimes stop taking your medicine?

Each item is scored 1 or 0. Scores on this scale successfully predicted blood pressure control at both 6 and 42 month follow-up, the correlations being 0.43 and 0.58 respectively. These questions are general ones which should be applicable to a wide range of compliance, and it will be interesting to see if they achieve similar success in other fields. Notice, however, that these questions implicitly assume that the patient has a correct understanding of the regimen, in that they do not probe the exact details of when the medicine is taken, etc. It is possible that predictive validity could be improved by inclusion of questions on these further topics.

In the pill and bottle count method the amount of medicine taken is assessed by seeing how many pills are left, or how much medicine remains in the bottle. Provided one knows how much there was to start with it is then possible to assess the amount which has been used. This can then be compared with the amount which should have been consumed, and an estimate of the patient's compliance obtained. This method also has its problems. First, patients can deceive the examiner by disposing of medicines other than swallowing them. Secondly, patients can forget to bring their medicine containers with them, and thus prevent the measure from being used. Thirdly the method usually assesses only the amount of medicine consumed, and provides no evidence on the scheduling of the doses. To obtain this information some form of patient report has to be used. This obviously lands one with the problems of the interview method.

Attempts to assess patients' intake of drugs by the measurement of blood and urine samples have at first glance great objectivity. However blood and urine levels of the drug-related samples are not usually monitored continuously. The usual procedure is for a sample to be taken on the occasion of a clinic visit. The validity of this assessment as a measure of long-term behaviour is clearly open to question, as with many substances the appropriate levels could be built up by taking the right doses for a day or two before attending the clinic. A second problem is that there is also the likelihood of individual differences in absorption and excretion rates. To the extent that this is so, it is possible for some of the better compliers to look worse on this measure than some who are complying less well. For any particular family of drugs it is necessary to establish the correlation between blood and urine test result and compliance. If this is not high then the method will be misleading in many cases. Other problems with this method are that it is not necessarily acceptable to all patients (which might distort the sample of patients available for assessment), and it is expensive. Because of the expense and lower acceptability to patients, the method is not really suitable in many research settings.

Mechanical devices to measure compliance have been used in clinical and analogue studies. They automatically provide some hard copy record of a patient's compliance-related behaviour. Thus Moulding (1962) invented a device which would automatically record when a medication container was opened. In an investigation of ophthalmological patients, Yee, Hahn and Christensen (1974) described a device which recorded whether or not a medication container had been opened in the previous hour or not, and in an analogue study Wilkins and Baddeley (1978) used a device which recorded the exact time at which compliant behaviour occurred. However, probably the most thorough use of such devices is in the researches conducted by Moulding and associates (Moulding, Knight, and Colson, 1967; Moulding, Onstad, and Sbarbaro, 1970; Moulding, 1971, 1974, 1979), and Norell and his co-workers, (Norell, 1979, 1981a,b, 1982a, 1985; Norell and Granstrom, 1980; Norell, Granstrom, and Wassen, 1980; Alfredsson and Norell, 1981; Grantsrom and Norell, 1983). The studies by Moulding and associates have mainly involved patients suffering from tuberculosis, whereas those by Norell and associates have been conducted with patients suffering from glaucoma, for whom pilocarpine drops had been prescribed. A major advantage of these mechanical recording devices is that they allow accurate assessment of the timing, (although not ncessarily the taking), of doses.

Direct observation of patients to assess whether they are complying or not has seldom if ever been used in practice, except of course where the compliant behaviour in question has been keeping an appointment.

In investigations into ways of reducing non-compliance some investigators have attempted to use outcome as a measure of compliance. The argument is that, given an effective treatment for a condition, those who are more compliant will on average respond better to treatment. The use of outcome as a measure of compliance has been used particularly in studies by compliance in obesity and hypertension. Thus, a group of obese patients with a high compliance rate will lose more weight than a group with a lower compliance rate. Putting people on scales and weighing them should therefore be an objective way of assessing relative compliance rates. Similarly drops in blood pressure should provide an objective indicator of relative compliance rates in groups of hypertensive patients. Because of individual differences in response to treatment the method is clearly suspect in the individual case. It also meets problems in comparisons between groups. These stem essentially from the fact that changes on the outcome variable might not be very responsive to changes in compliance. For instance if the change in compliance needed for a measurabe change in the outcome variable is 25 per cent then the method will be incapable of detecting quite large differences in compliance. That this must sometimes happen is demonstrated by the fact that sometimes quite large proportions of patients who have complied well with a treatment regimen do not show a satisfactory therapeutic response. Thus, for example, Lowenthal, Briggs, Mutterperl, Adelman and Creditor (1976) and Sackett (1979) reported that approximately 60 per cent of patients taking their medicines properly did not achieve target blood pressure levels. In the same studies 16 and 28 per cent, respectively, of those who did not comply well did achieve the required blood pressure level. All of this should lead to caution in the use of outcome as a measure of compliance.

Some investigators have used physician's judgement of whether the patient is complying or not as a criterion. This method has never been widely used and is now out of favour because of its low validity. Investigation has shown that physicians are poor judges of whether or not their patients are complying (Brody, 1980; Granstrom and Norell, 1983; Caron, 1985). A good example of this is presented in the investigation by Brody, who found that the physicians failed to identify the 79 per cent of their patients who were underconsuming regular medications.

Caron (1985) has reported on the relative frequency with which these different methods of assessing compliance were used in a sample of studies reported between 1977 and 1983. Sixty-six per cent of these investigations used only one method of assessing compliance, and of these two-thirds relied on patients' report as their measure. The next most frequent measure was outcome which was used in 9 per cent of these studies. In the group of studies as a whole, i.e. both those which used only one measure and those which used two or more measures of compliance, patients' report was used in 68 per cent; outcome in 40 per cent; direct observation (appointment keeping/drop-out), in 14 per cent; pill count in 12 per cent; mechanical device in 10 per cent; and blood or urine test in 6 per cent.

In practice the easiest ways of assessing compliance are patients' report and pill counts. Patients' report has the merit of being easy to obtain, and, as has been mentioned earlier, in the version used by Morisky *et al.* (1986) can have considerable long-term predictive validity. In general patients' report correlates significantly with other measures of compliance. Pill counts also correlate significantly with other measures of measuring compliance. This can be seen in Table 4.1, which provides a summary of studies of the correlations between different measures of assessing compliance. Where a study did not report a correlation coefficient, but provided information in the appropriate form the correlation has been assessed by calculating a Phi coefficient.

Another way of assessing the different methods is to compare the degree of non-compliance reported for different methods when these are used in the same study. Table 4.2 provides a summary of studies which compared estimates of non-compliance based on patients' report with estimates based on more objective methods such as pill-counts or blood or urine tests. It can be seen that the levels of non-compliance as judged by the more objective methods are higher than those based on patients' report.

Other studies supporting the conclusion that objective methods yield higher estimates of non-compliance include those of Chaves (1960), Francis, Korsch and Morris (1969), Moulding *et al.* (1970), Rickels and Briscoe (1970), and Sheiner, Rosenberg, Marathe and Peck (1974).

It also appears to be true that blood and urine tests lead to higher estimates of non-compliance than do pill-counts. For example, Bergman and Werner (1963) reported that non-compliance among patients taking penicillin was 82 per cent as judged by pill-count and 92 per cent as judged by urine test. Similarly, Leistyna and Macaulay (1966); and Roth, Caron and Hsi (1970) have reported results showing that pill counts yield lower estimates of non-compliance.

Table 4.1: Relationships between different methods for measuring compliance

Investigation	Patients	r	p
1. Patients' report versus:			
(a) Pill and bottle counts			
Park and Lipman (1964)	Depressed	0.23	< 0.05
Roth (1979)	Peptic ulcer	0.42	< 0.05
Sackett (1979)	Hypertensive	0.43	< 0.05
Haynes et al. (1980b)	Hypertensive	0.74	< 0.05
Inui et al. (1980)	Hypertensive	0.43	< 0.05
(b) Blood test			
Becker et al. (1978)	Asthmatic	0.91	< 0.05
(c) Mechanical device			
Norell (1981)	Ophthalmic	0.38	< 0.05
Taylor et al. (1983)	Hypertensive	0.88	< 0.05
Hoelscher et al. (1986)	Hypertensive	0.64–0.89	< 0.001
(d) Physician's estimate			
Norell (1981)	Ophthalmic	− 0.10	n.s.
Cochran (1984)	Affective	(a) − 0.09	n.s.
		(b) 0.40	< 0.05
		(c) 0.34	n.s.
(e) Outcome			
Morisky et al. (1986)	Hypertensive		
	(a) 6 months	0.43	< 0.01
	(b) 42 months	0.58	< 0.01
2. Physician's estimate versus:			
(a) Pill and bottle counts			
Caron and Roth (1968)	Peptic ulcer	0.01	n.s.
Roth (1979)	Peptic ulcer	0.48	< 0.05
(b) Objective measures			
Mushlin and Appel (1977)	Cardiac	0.27	< 0.05
Norell (1981)	Ophthalmic	(a) 0.19	n.s.
		(b) 0.30	< 0.05
3. Pill and bottle count versus:			
Blood or urine test			
Leistyna et al. (1966)	Pediatric	0.62	< 0.05
Haynes et al. (1980b)	Hypertensive		
(a) blood test		(a) 0.49	< 0.05
		(b) 0.35	< 0.05
(b) urine test		(a) 0.41	< 0.05
		(b) 0.19	< 0.05
Caron (1985)	Peptic ulcer	0.80	< 0.05

Table 4.2: Comparisons of the magnitude of patients'
non-compliance as assessed by patients' own report and by
more objective methods

| Investigation | Per cent *not* complying as assessed by: | |
	Patients' report	More objective method
Feinstein *et al.* (1959)	27	45
Bergman and Werner (1963)	17	82
Park and Lipman (1964)	15	51
Preston and Miller (1964)	4	28
Gordis (1969)	(a) 27	58
	(b) 31	67
Hecht (1974)	21	47
Sackett (1979)	22	50
Inui *et al.* (1980)	39	62
Norell (1981)	14	49

THE MAGNITUDE OF THE PROBLEM

From what has already been presented it will be obvious to the
reader that any simple statement of the magnitude of the
problem of patients' non-compliance will be impossible. The
percentage judged as non-compliant will vary with the criterion
used and the method of measurement. For example, it would
appear from the data summarised in Table 4.2 that if non-
compliance is assessed by patients' report the percentage judged
non-compliant will be less than half of what it would be if more
objective methods are used. It is also likely that if the criterion
for judging a patient to be compliant is set at 100 per cent
compliance with the prescribed regimen then this will result in
higher rates of non-compliance than if the criterion is set at 80
per cent compliance with that regimen. In addition to this there
will be the usual variation to be expected from differences
between samples, length of investigation and so on.

These qualifications should be borne in mind when looking
at Table 4.3, which summarises three reviews of studies reporting percentages of patients judged compliant. The data reported
by Ley (1976) were derived from investigations reported in
1969 or earlier, whereas the Department of Health and Human
Welfare data are derived from studies reported in 1970 or later.

Table 4.3: Patients' non-compliance with advice

Area of advice	Mean percentage non-compliant in review by:		
	Ley (1976, 1978)	Department of Health Education and Welfare (1979)	Sackett and Snow (1979)
(a) Medication			
Anti-tubercular	38.5	42.0	41.0
Antiobiotic	49.0	47.7	—
Cardiovascular	—	39.3	38.7
Miscellaneous	48.0	52.0	42.5
Multiple drug regimen	—	60.0	—
Psychiatric	38.6	42.0	52.0
All medications	43.4	48.2	40.9
(b) Attendance at clinics			
Obesity	47.7	—	—
Other	—	—	46.6
(c) Diet			
Various	49.4	—	—
(d) Other advice			
Miscellaneous	54.6	—	57.7

The review by Sackett and Snow (1979) included only studies which these authors considered to be methodologically superior. Data from Ley (1978) on attendance at obesity clinics are also included in the table.

Considering the difficulties besetting any attempt to arrive at overall figures for non-compliance it is of some interest to note that for medications as a whole there is reasonable congruence on the percentage of patients not taking their medicines properly. Further, within subcategories there is good agreement between the reviews of Ley (1976) and the Department of Health, Education and Welfare (1979). Because the review by Sackett and Snow (1979) included a smaller number of studies means for subcategories for their data are based on very small numbers of studies indeed. Hence the apparent discrepancies between these data and those of the other two reviews should not be taken too seriously.

As well as reviews of compliance by patients in general there have been a number of reviews of patients in particular diagnostic groupings, e.g. hypertension (Haynes, Mattson and

Engebretson, 1980a; Haynes, Mattson, Chobanian, Dunbar, Engebretson, Garrity, Leventhal, Levine and Levy, 1982; Luscher, Vetter, Siegenthaler and Vetter, 1985). Such reviews of compliance in particular diagnostic groups show that non-compliance is a phenomenon affecting all groups, and that its magnitude seems to be similar throughout these groups. Two groups which are of special interest, because it might be thought that there would be special factors likely to increase non-compliance amongst their members, are the elderly and psychiatric patients. It is therefore worthwhile to consider these groups in more detail.

COMPLIANCE OF ELDERLY PATIENTS

The aged might be less compliant on account of poorer sensory acuity, poorer memory, and greater likelihood of living alone. Indeed there is some evidence that poorer visual acuity and muscular strength can lead to great difficulties in actually gaining access to their medications. For example in one sample of elderly people Kendrick and Bayne (1982) found that 13 per cent could not open flip-top pill containers, 53 per cent had difficulty with palm-turned caps, and nearly two-thirds had difficulty with caps which required the lining up of two arrows. A further finding was that 58 per cent could not discriminate between pills of differing shades of yellow. These findings make the examination of non-compliance rates in the elderly a matter of some interest.

A further factor that makes this a problem of some concern is that the elderly are proportionately heavy consumers of medication. Thus, for example, in the USA they make up 11 per cent of the population but consume 25–30 per cent of prescriptions (Olins, 1985), and average, including repeats, some 13 prescriptions a year (Millstein, 1985). In addition, 86 per cent of people over age 65 have one or more chronic conditions, requiring long-term medication (Richardson, 1986).

Several studies of compliance in the elderly are therefore summarised in Table 4.4.

It can be seen that estimates of compliance rates in the elderly range widely as they do in other age groups. Mean compliance in these investigations is 51 per cent. This compares favourably with the studies summarised in Table 4.3. These data

63

Table 4.4: Non-compliance in the elderly

Investigation	Patients	Age	Method of assessing compliance	Percentage non-compliant
Schwartz et al. (1962)	178 outpatients	60+	Interview	59
Law and Chalmers (1976)	132 general practice	75+	Interview and pill count	30
MacDonald et al. (1977)	60 recently discharged	'Aged'	Pill count	(a) 1 week 67 (b) 6 weeks 77
Crome et al. (1980)	51 inpatients	'Aged'	Pill count	67
Spriet et al. (1980)	1662 outpatients	'Aged'	Pill count	38
Cooper et al. (1982)	111 community sample	60+	Interview	43
Crome et al. (1982)	38 recently discharged patients	'Aged'	Pill count	66
German et al. (1982)	139 recently discharged patients	65+	Interview	54
Smith and Andrews (1983)	30 recently discharged patients	65+	Pill count	8
Edwards and Pathy (1984)	44 discharged patients	65+	Pill count	57

therefore offer no evidence of greater non-compliance in the elderly.

This conclusion is supported by the summary of Haynes, Taylor and Sackett (1979) who found no consistent relationship between age and compliance. It is also well exemplified in the findings of the investigation by German, Klein, McPhee and Smith (1982) in which a large sample of patients discharged from hospital on various medication regimens reported a compliance rate of 49 per cent in 372 patients under aged 65, whereas 46 per cent of 171 patients aged 65 and over were compliant with their treatment. Similarly, Meagher, O'Brien, and O'Malley (1985) reported that 83 per cent of hypertensive patients in the 60–69 age group were still active participants in the treatment programme after two years, compared to 81–85 per cent of younger age groups.

Thus non-compliance is a problem in the treatment of the elderly as well as in the treatment of younger groups, but it does not seem to be a significantly greater problem. Nevertheless the difficulties experienced by some of the elderly with medicine containers, referred to above, obviously need attention.

COMPLIANCE OF PSYCHIATRIC PATIENTS

Psychiatric patients are another group in which it might be expected that non-compliance would be a particular problem. This would be expected to be particularly true of psychotic patients. However, it can be seen in Table 4.3 that the reviews by Ley (1976) and the Department of Health, Education and Welfare (1979) do not support this view. In those reviews mean non-compliance rates among psychiatric patients were 39 and 42 per cent respectively, compared with overall rates of 43 and 48 per cent in these two reviews. Thus these data do not support the view that there will be a more serious non-compliance problem in the case of psychiatric patients. Nevertheless, it is clearly possible that patients in certain diagnostic categories will have particular problems in complying with advice about medication. The two diagnostic categories which have received most attention in this regard are schizophrenia, and major affective disorder.

Barofsky and Connelly (1983) reviewed the literature on compliance among schizophrenic patients in the community. It was found that the mean non-compliance rate for oral medications was 46.3 per cent, while for long acting phenothiazines, given by injection, it was 17.2 per cent.

Compliance with lithium regimens by outpatients suffering from bipolar affective disorders has been reviewed by Cochran (1986). Mean percentage non-compliant was found to be 29.3 per cent. These results for psychiatric patients are summarised in Table 4.5.

Table 4.5: Non-compliance in psychiatric patients

Reviewer	Type of patient	Mean percentage non-compliant
Ley (1976)	Various	38.6
Dept. of Health, Education and Welfare (1979)	Various	42.0
Barofsky and Connelly (1983)	Schizophrenic	46.3
Cochran (1986)	Bipolar affective	29.3

As in the case of elderly patients it emerges that there is a problem, but also as in the case of elderly patients it would appear that the problem is of the same magnitude as for patients in general.

COSTS OF NON-COMPLIANCE

The US Department of Health and Human Services (1980) provided estimates of the costs of non-compliance with regimens for ten common prescription drugs. The drugs involved were: ampicillins, benzodiazepines, cimetidine, clofibrate, digoxin, methoxsalen, propoxyphene, phenytoin, thiazides and warfarin. The possible consequences of non-compliance considered were the need for a further prescription; extra visits to the doctor; extra time off work; and the need for hospitalisation. The costs of these individual outcomes, in 1979 US dollars, were estimated as follows:

(a) extra prescription: 7 dollars;
(b) visit to doctor: 15 dollars;
(c) day in hospital: 250 dollars;
(d) workday lost: 45 dollars.

It was further estimated that, in the USA, there would be

some 75 million prescriptions per year for these drugs, in which non-compliance could cause problems. Finally it was assumed that non-compliance rates woud be about 40 per cent. Given these figures it was possible to estimate the costs of non-compliance. The results of this exercise are shown in Table 4.6.

Table 4.6: Estimated costs of non-compliance with regimens for ten common drug classes

Source of cost	Estimated occurrence (%)	Estimated cost (1979) (millions of US dollars)
Unnecessary prescription refill	10.0–20.0	21.0–42.0
One additional physician visit	5.0–10.0	22.5–45.0
One additional workday lost	5.0–10.0	67.5–135.0
Two additional workdays lost	5.0–10.0	135.0–270.0
Hospitalisation:		
One day	0.25–0.5	18.75–37.5
Two days	0.50–1.0	75.0–150.0
Three days	0.25–0.5	56.26–112.5
Total		396.0–792.0

Other research has tackled the problem from a slightly different perspective. For example, McKenney and Harrison (1976) interviewed all patients admitted to a general ward in a large teaching hospital during a two-month period to ascertain the reasons for admission. In this sample of 216 patients, it was found that in 10 per cent of cases admission was the result of non-compliance with the medication regimen. Ausburn (1981) also assessed reasons for admission to medical wards among a sample of 205 patients and found that in 20 per cent of cases admission was probably, and in a further 5 per cent of cases was possibly related to non-compliance. Thus between a tenth and a quarter of medical inpatient beds were occupied by patients who were in hospital because of non-compliance. These findings also suggest that non-compliance is expensive.

As well as these financial costs there are of course the great human costs to patients and their families in terms of suffering and inconvenience.

CORRELATES OF NON-COMPLIANCE

In their major review and annotated bibliography of the compliance literature Haynes *et al.* (1979) summarised studies of the relationships between compliance and patient, disease, regimen, and physician–patient interaction characteristics. Over 100 patient characteristics, 13 disease, 13 regimen, and 49 physician–patient interaction characteristics had been studied. For most of the patient characteristics the commonest finding was that the majority of studies showed no association with compliance. Exceptions to this generalisation included:

(a) Health Belief Model variables (perceived variability, seriousness of illness, effectiveness of treatment and costs and barriers);
(b) influence of friends and family;
(c) compliance with other aspects of the regimen.

It was also found that for all but one of the disease characteristics studied the commonest finding was that there was no association with compliance, and the exception was a characteristic which had only been investigated in two studies.

In the case of regimen characteristics, the ones which did show a relationship to compliance were:

(a) duration of therapy;
(b) complexity of regimen as assessed by the number of drugs or treatments involved.

Further many of the studies which failed to find a relationship between duration of treatment and compliance were cross-sectional in nature. Studies which followed a cohort of patients longitudinally overwhelmingly report that compliance decreases with increasing duration of treatment.

Most features of the interaction between patient and therapist which have been investigated have been studied in too few studies for any generalisation to be made. However, the following characteristics of the interaction had been shown to be associated with compliance:

(a) patients' satisfaction;
(b) patients' expectations being met;
(c) level of supervision by the therapist.

Table 4.7 summarises these results.

In general later research has supported these findings. In the case of the Health Belief Model variables the case for their

Table 4.7: Some correlates of compliance

Correlate	Number of studies showing stated association with compliance		
	Positive	No difference	Negative
Health Belief Model variables:			
Vulnerability	15	3	1
Seriousness	10	7	2
Efficacy of treatment	8	8	0
Compliance with other aspects of regimen	11	3	0
Influence of family and friends	19	10	1
Patient satisfaction	8	0	0
Patients' expectations met	6	0	0
Level of supervision	6	0	0
Duration of therapy	1	9	13
Complexity of regimen	2	3	9

being important determinants of compliance now looks considerably stronger. A series of reviews have shown that these variables are not only correlated with current compliance (Becker, 1976, 1979; Gochman and Parcel, 1982; King, 1983), but also that they predict future compliance (Janz and Becker, 1984). This latter finding is particularly important in that any association found between *current* compliance and variables such as those in the Health Belief Model could arise because:

(a) the beliefs have a causal effect on compliance;
(b) the beliefs are affected by the patient's compliance;
(c) common factors affect both beliefs and compliance.

The best way to distinguish between these possibilities is to conduct prospective studies, in which beliefs are measured before compliance has or has not occurred, and see how well the beliefs predict later compliance. Although there are some studies which have found that health beliefs do not predict future compliance, e.g. Becker, Maiman, Kirscht, Haefner, Drachman and Taylor (1979); Smith, Ley, Seale and Shaw (1987), the majority of studies show that the beliefs have predictive validity.

Janz and Becker (1984) have reviewed 46 studies of health beliefs. Of these 28 were retrospective and 18 were prospective investigations. The model was found to have a high success rate. Susceptibility showed the appropriate relationship in 81 per cent of studies; severity, in 65 per cent; efficacy of treatment and other benefits, in 78 per cent; and barriers, in 89 per cent. Further, it was found that these associations were just as frequently found in the prospective as in the retrospective studies.

Finally, because it is easy to remedy, it is worth making special mention of the effects of length of time spent waiting to see the doctor. A good example of this can be found in the study by Geersten, Gray, and Ward (1973). These investigators found that whereas 67 per cent of patients who had waited 30 minutes or less to see the doctor were compliant, only 48 per cent of those who had waited between 31 and 59 minutes, and only 31 per cent of those who had waited more than an hour were compliant with advice. In this study the majority of patients had had to wait more than 30 minutes and a third had had to wait over an hour.

SUMMARY

This chapter has provided a brief review of the problem of patients' non-compliance with advice. The different methods for assessing compliance were reviewed and it was shown that the most popular method, patients' report, correlates significantly with other methods of measurement. Further these other methods tend to correlate significantly with one another as well. The two methods of assessing compliance which seem to be most problematical are the use of therapeutic outcome as a measure and the use of the clinician's guess as to whether the patient is complying or not.

Different methods of measurement tend to produce different estimates of the frequency of non-compliance, which is usually judged lowest by patients' report, somewhat higher by pill counts, and higher still by blood and urine tests.

As assessed by various mixtures of these measures the average percentage of patients likely to be non-compliant seems to be between 40 and 50 per cent, but the range of percentages non-compliant is considerable. For example in the case of studies of non-compliance with medication regimens it is from 8 to 95 per cent.

Non-compliance costs a great deal of money. In 1979 US dollars the costs in the USA of non-compliance with ten common classes of prescribed medications were estimated to be between 396 and 792 million dollars. Also, non-compliance with medication regimens is a significant cause of hospital admission.

Factors shown to be associated with non-compliance include Health Belief Model variables; patient satisfaction; the meeting of patients' expectations; the duration and complexity of the regimen; the level of supervision provided; and the influence of family and friends.

The various methods for decreasing non-compliance and their effectiveness will be discussed in later chapters. It will now be profitable to examine the relationships between understanding, memory, satisfaction, and compliance.

Relationships Between Understanding, Memory, Satisfaction and Compliance

INTRODUCTION

Having reviewed the topics of patients' satisfaction, understanding, memory and compliance it is time to consider the interrelationships of these variables. A model much concerned with these interrelationships is the Cognitive Model (Ley, 1977; 1982b,c), which predicts that there will be significant correlations between understanding, memory, satisfaction, and compliance. Understanding will have direct effects on memory, satisfaction and compliance, and, through its effect on satisfaction, an additional indirect effect on compliance. Similarly memory will affect compliance directly and also exert an indirect effect through its effect on satisfaction. Finally satisfaction will have a direct effect on compliance. These predicted relationships are shown in Figure 5.1.

In the studies to be summarised the definition of understanding has varied, as has its method of assessment. Definitions have included:

    (a) the patient's knowledge of the details of the treatment regimen;
    (b) the patient's knowledge of the rationale of treatment;
    (c) the patient's knowledge of the illness;
    (d) mixtures of the above.

These different types of understanding might well have different effects on compliance. It would be expected that the first would be a necessary condition for compliance. If the patient does not know the details of the treatment regimen then

Figure 5.1: The hypothesised relationships between understanding, memory, satisfaction, and compliance

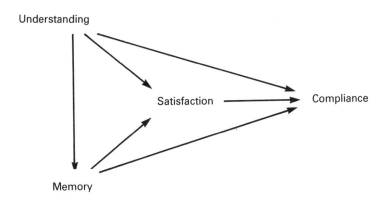

any compliance would be the result of either chance or base-rate medicine taking behaviours. The concept of base-rate medicine taking behaviours is simply that it is possible that people have a general idea of how often tablets should be taken. Let us suppose that, in the absence of any other information, a proportion of people think that tablets should be taken four times a day. If by chance that is the frequency with which a particular tablet should be taken, then those people, even though they have not remembered or understood the details of the regimen, will be taking their tablet with the correct frequency. Of course if the tablet is one which should be taken three times a day then such people will get the frequency wrong.

The other two types of understanding, i.e. knowledge of the rationale of treatment and knowledge of the illness, would be expected to affect compliance, but they are not necessary conditions for compliance in the way that knowledge of the treatment regimen is. Unfortunately there are not enough investigations of pure examples of these different types of understanding to make any conclusive comparisons between them possible. Despite this it is definitely known that non-compliance can sometimes remain completely unaffected in conditions where there is no doubt that patients have reasonably complete understanding in all three areas (Sackett *et al.*, 1975).

There have also been differences between studies in the way in which memory has been assessed. Some studies have used the free recall method, and others a multiple choice test. Definitions of satisfaction have included both satisfaction with the consult-ation as a whole and satisfaction with communications. Finally compliance has been variously assessed in the different studies. Methods have included patients' own reports and pill counts. Once more there are not enough studies available for it to be possible to assess the effects of these varying definitions and methods of measurement.

RELATIONSHIP BETWEEN UNDERSTANDING AND MEMORY, SATISFACTION, AND COMPLIANCE

Studies which have provided data on these relationships are summarised in Table 5.1. In some of these investigations, and in some of those to be reported later, results were not presented in the form of a correlation coefficient, but gave sufficient detail for Eta or Phi to be calculated. In these cases the value of Eta or Phi has been recorded as the correlation coefficient. The calculation of the mean correlation coefficients recorded was made using the z-tranformations of the correlations reported in the tables.

It can be seen that the mean correlation between understand-ing and memory is 0.34; between understanding and satisfac-tion 0.58; and between understanding and compliance it is 0.36. Thus these results support the predictions made from the model.

RELATIONSHIP BETWEEN MEMORY AND SATISFACTION AND COMPLIANCE

Table 5.2 summarises the relevant data and shows that, as predicted, memory correlates with both satisfaction and compli-ance, the mean correlations being 0.20 and 0.29 respectively.

RELATIONSHIP BETWEEN SATISFACTION AND COMPLIANCE

A number of studies offering evidence concerning the magni-tude of this relationship were found. These are summarised in Table 5.3, where it can be seen that the mean correlation between satisfaction and compliance is 0.26.

Table 5.1: Relationships between understanding and memory, satisfaction and compliance

Investigation		Correlation coefficient	Mean correlation
(a) Understanding and memory			*0.34*
Ley *et al.* (1972)		0.38	
Bradshaw *et al.* (1975)	(a)	0.17	
	(b)	0.41	
	(c)	0.45	
Ley *et al.* (1979)		0.33	
Eaton and Holloway (1980)		0.28	
Ley (1982c)		0.36	
(b) Understanding and satisfaction			*0.58*
Ley, Skilbeck and Tulips (1975b)		0.68	
Ley, Swinson *et al.* (1975)		0.45	
Ley *et al.* (1976a)		0.34	
Ley *et al.* (1976b)	(a)	0.69	
	(b)	0.64	
(c) Understanding and compliance			*0.36*
Watkins *et al.* (1967)		0.44	
Tagliacozzo and Ima (1970)	(a)	0.22	
	(b)	0.39	
Kincey *et al.* (1975)		0.23	
Ley *et al.* (1975a)		0.35	
Ley, Skilbeck and Tulips (1975b)		0.20	
Sackett *et al.* (1975)		0.08	
Ley *et al.* (1976b)	(a)	0.31	
	(b)	0.52	
Parkin *et al.* (1976)		0.73	
De Wet and Hollingshead (1980)		0.36	
German *et al.* (1982)		0.02	
Smith *et al.* (1986)	(a)	0.43	
	(b)	0.48	

Table 5.2: Relationships between memory and satisfaction and compliance

Investigation	Correlation coefficient	Mean correlation
(a) Memory and satisfaction		*0.20*
Bertakis (1977)	0.28	
Romm and Hulka (1979)	0.20	
Brody (1980)	0.28	
Bartlett *et al.* (1984)	0.02	
(b) Memory and compliance		*0.29*
Ley *et al.* (1974)	0.29	
Bartlett *et al.* (1984)	0.29	

Table 5.3: Relationship between satisfaction and compliance

Investigation		Correlation coefficient	Mean correlation
Satisfaction and compliance			*0.26*
Francis *et al.* (1969)		0.24	
Geersten *et al.* (1973)		0.07	
Ley *et al.* (1975b)		0.19	
Ley *et al.* (1976b)	(a)	0.24	
	(b)	0.67	
Falvo *et al.* (1980)	(a)	0.23	
	(b)	0.24	
Wartman *et al.* (1983)		−0.13	
Bartlett *et al.* (1984)		0.24	
Smith *et al.* (1986)	(a)	0.35	
	(b)	0.42	

SUMMARY

All of the relationships predicted by the Cognitive Model are supported by the mean correlations obtained. Understanding, memory, satisfaction and compliance show the appropriate interrelationships. It should be noted, however, that some studies have found no relationship between the relevant variables, and secondly that the mean correlations reported are not very high. The exception to this being the mean correlation between understanding and satisfaction.

What are the implications of these correlations? Rosenthal and Rubin (1982) have proposed a method for the interpretation of correlations, which they have called the Behavioral Effect Size Display. It has been argued by Ley (1986) that this method can be applied to correlations such as those reported above. (The reader interested in the mechanics of this method is referred to these two papers.) Using the method we can estimate, for example, that among patients with adequate comprehension, on average, 67 per cent will have adequate memory of what they have been told; 79 per cent will feel satisfied with the communications aspect of the consultation; and 68 per cent will show adequate compliance. Corresponding percentages for those not having adequate comprehension would be 33 per cent with adequate recall; 21 per cent satisfied; and 32 per cent compliant. So even though the correlations are small in magnitude they imply differences which are large enough to be of interest in practical clinical situations. Some further uses of these data will be discussed in later chapters.

A further implication is of course that it should be possible to achieve worthwhile gains in patients' satisfaction and compliance by improving understanding and memory. Later chapters will examine some of the methods for increasing comprehension and memory and the effects of such increases on satisfaction and compliance.

6

Techniques for Increasing Patients' Recall and Understanding

INTRODUCTION

Several investigations have reported on the effectiveness of various strategies for improving patients' recall. These researches have attempted either to improve recall of particular content or to increase the overall amount recalled. The recall of content has been achieved by the use of primacy effects and by stressing the importance of selected portions of the message, but there is relatively little research on these topics. There is much more research into ways of increasing the total amount recalled. Methods for achieving this objective have included (a) simplification of the information, (b) the use of explicit categorisation, (c) repetition, and (d) the use of specific rather than general advice statements.

Repeating the information about appointments in the form of telephoned and posted reminders has also been used to reduce forgetting of their time and place. This research has concentrated on the effects of reminders on compliance in appointment keeping, and has, perhaps with good reason, assumed that their effects in increasing recall can be taken for granted.

The effectiveness of 'mechanical aids' to memory has also been investigated. These studies have concentrated on compliance in medicine taking as the criterion of success, and, as in the case of reminders, it has been taken for granted that their use will reduce forgetting.

In this chapter attention will be paid to those studies which have studied these techniques in relation to oral presentation of material. The research involving improvement of recall of written materials will be considered in later chapters after the usefulness of written information has been discussed.

IMPROVING RECALL OF PARTICULAR CONTENT

In the earlier discussion of factors related to how much patients recall of what they are told there was a review of the evidence showing that patients recall best what they are told first. Ley (1972b) argued that this primacy effect could be used to increase recall of instruction and advice statements, which in the study of Ley and Spelman (1965) had been poorly recalled. Accordingly, a series of outpatients, attending the same clinic as that involved in the earlier report, were presented with instructions and advice before being given other information such as their diagnosis, explanation of symptoms and the like. Mean recall of instructions and advice was 86 per cent in this group, compared with mean recall of 50 per cent in the group who did not receive instructions and advice first.

Ley also arranged for another group of outpatients to be given the information in the usual order but with the importance of remembering instructions and advice stressed just before their presentation. In this condition mean recall of instructions and advice increased to 65 per cent. It is clear that this experiment was marred by not arranging for random assignment of patients to the three conditions. Although there were practical constraints which made this impossible, and although Ley showed that the three samples were similar in most important respects, this lack of randomisation remains a problem. It is obviously less so in the case of the primacy effect which is well supported in other experiments involving recall of medical information, than in the case of stressing importance, which has received virtually no research attention.

Another finding of this research was that although recall of instructions and advice appeared to be improved there was no change in the overall proportion recalled. As recall of instructions and advice increased so recall of diagnostic and other statements declined. Attention was therefore directed to the discovery of methods for increasing the total percentage remembered.

INCREASING THE AMOUNT RECALLED

Simplification

The simplification technique is merely the use of shorter words and shorter sentences. With this shortening of word and sentence length the material presented becomes easier to understand and thus more meaningful to the patient. Most research using this technique has involved written information, and this will be described later. However, one study has used oral presentation of the information.

This investigation by Bradshaw *et al.* (1975) found that recall of dietary advice by obese women was enhanced when the advice was recast in shorter words and shorter sentences. In the ordinary condition mean recall of the advice was 27 per cent, increasing to 40 per cent when the material was simplified. As will be seen later there is ample confirmation of the benefits of simplification in studies using written materials.

Explicit categorisation

This technique, loosely based on the finding that categorisation has been found to aid recall in laboratory studies of memory, was first described by Ley *et al.* (1973). The technique consists of the clinician telling the patient what categories of information are to be provided, and then presenting the information category by category. For example;

'Now I am going to tell you:
What is wrong with you;
What tests and investigations will be necessary;
What the treatment will be;
What you must do to help yourself get better;
and what the outcome will be.

First, what is wrong — I think you've got bronchitis.
Secondly, what tests and investigations are necessary — you will have to have an X-ray, and a blood test to make sure.
Thirdly, what the treatment will be — I'll give you an antibiotic to take. Take it on an empty stomach, say at least one hour before a meal, and at least two hours after your last meal. Take it with a glass of water, never with milk, because milk will stop it working. Antacid tablets will also destroy its effectiveness. Make sure you take the full course of tablets.
Fourthly, what you must do to help yourself — don't go out in the fog, and don't smoke. Stay off work for a few days. Come

and see me at this time next week.

Lastly, what I think the outcome will be, you should be better in about a week, and can go back to work then.'

Ley *et al.* described an analogue and a clinical investigation using this technique. In the analogue study university students were randomly assigned to recalling 15 statements. In the normal condition mean recall was 43 per cent of the 15 statements presented, while in the explicitly categorised condition it rose to 61 per cent. The clinical study was conducted with a series of 40 consecutive new attenders in a general practice, who were randomly assigned to the normal presentation or to an explicitly categorised method of presentation. In the normal condition mean recall was 50 per cent, increasing to 64 per cent when explicit categorisation was used.

Further evidence for the effectiveness of the technique in analogue studies was provided by Ley (1979a), who reported the results of six further investigations using various amounts of information about different diagnoses. In all six studies mean recall was higher in the explicitly categorised condition. Average mean recall in the normal condition was 36 per cent and this rose to 50 per cent when explicit categorisation was used.

Reynolds, Sanson-Fisher, Poole, Harker and Byrne (1981), in a study conducted in an oncology clinic, also used a variant of this technique to increase patients' recall. The technique varied from that used by Ley and his collaborators in that the opening statement was changed so as to inform the patient that they would have to specify which categories of information they would like to have. The wording was as follows.

'If you would like to know I will tell you: (1) what is wrong with you and what the diagnosis is; (2) what the treatment will be' etc. As each category was re-announced the patient had to indicate whether the information was required or not. Patients in the group receiving explicitly categorised material also received a written copy of the information presented to them. Control patients were given nothing in writing. Recall was assessed at follow-ups at 5 days and 6 weeks later. Control patients were asked at these interviews about the categories of information they wanted. At five-day follow-up control patients recalled on average 48 per cent, compared with the 66 per cent recalled by the experimental group. At six weeks the figures were 55 per cent and 64 per cent respectively. Further analyses showed that the experimental group had received a much higher average number of statements than the control group (28.1 compared with 18.2). This difference and the provision of written information to the explicit categorisation group make interpretation of this study difficult. However it raises the intriguing possibility that explicit categorisation might, in some circumstances, have a major effect on the amount of information the clinician presents.

Repetition

It is clear that the use of the explicit categorisation technique takes some time. Indeed in the time needed to use it, it would be possible to repeat everything to the patient, or alternatively have the patient repeat everything back.

Kupst *et al.* (1975) assessed the effectiveness of both these techniques. Patients were assigned, in such a way as to control for (a) severity of illness, and (b) which physician was seen, to a single presentation of the information, to having it repeated by the physician, or to having to repeat it themselves. Immediate mean recall was 76 per cent for the single presentation, 90 per cent when the physician repeated the material, and 91 per cent when the patient did so. The advantage shown in the repetition conditions persisted at one month follow-up when recall was tested by postal questionnaire.

Further evidence of the benefits of having the patient repeat back what is said is provided by Bertakis (1977). This investigator compared recall of patients exposed to a single presentation of information, with recall by patients who had to repeat back what they had been told. Two separate series of 50 patients were involved and thus assignment to conditions was not random. After the usual single presentation mean recall was 62 per cent of the 13 or so statements presented. In the repetition condition it was 83 per cent of the average of 11.5 statements made by the doctor.

Repetition also seems to increase recall in analogue studies. Ley (1979a) reported the average mean recall in six studies increased from 33 per cent to 47 per cent when the information was repeated by the presenter. However, the effect in these analogue studies was not a very robust one, in that in one experiment it was not found at all, and in several others the increase was not significant.

Use of specific advice statements

During the earlier mentioned research into the perceived importance of different categories of medical statements it happened that by mistake the lists of statements studied included some which were quite similar to others included in the list. In each case one of the pair of statements was more specific in its meaning, the other being more general. The statements and perceptions of their importance are shown in Table 6.1, where it will be seen that, except in the case of the statement about further visits, the more specific of the pair received higher ratings of importance.

Table 6.1: The rated importance of some specifically and generally phrased advice statements

Statement	Number of times specific version judged more important (%)	p
Stop smoking		
Cut down the amount you smoke	77	<0.01
You must lose two stone in weight		
You must lose weight	72	<0.01
Take two full weeks holiday a year		
You need regular holidays	70	<0.01
I will see you again in two weeks		
I shall want to see you again soon	44	n.s.

Bradshaw *et al.* (1975) argued that if specific statements were judged more important, and if important statements were more likely to be recalled, then it should follow that re-phrasing advice statements in a more specific form would increase the probability of their being recalled. Accordingly the sample of obese women, referred to above, were presented with dietary advice in either general or specific form. When the statements were in general form 16 per cent were recalled, while in the specific form 51 per cent were recalled. Again, as will be seen below, research using material presented in written form confirms this finding.

A mixture of these techniques

Ley *et al.* (1976b) investigated the effectiveness of a package of these techniques in a general practice setting. A brief manual containing a description of the use of primacy and importance effects, simplification, explicit categorisation, repetition, and specific statements was prepared. The manual also contained a summary of the evidence on which each suggested technique was based. Patients' recall of what their doctors had said was assessed in a baseline phase before any of the four doctors involved had read the manual or were aware of the techniques involved.

After this baseline assessment period, the doctors read the manual and tried to put its suggestions into effect. Table 6.2 shows the results of this study. It can be seen that the patients of all four doctors showed increased recall in the period after the doctors had read the manual. Recall in the baseline condition ranged across doctors from 52 to 59 per cent, and in the experimental phase, from 61 to 80 per cent. Table 6.2 also summarises the effectiveness of the other memory-enhancing techniques described above.

Table 6.2: Effectiveness of memory-enhancing techniques in increasing recall of orally presented medical information

Investigation	Technique	Percentage Recalled		
		Control	Experimental	p
Clinical studies				
Ley (1972b)	Primacy	50	86	<0.01
	Stressed importance		65	<0.06
Bradshaw *et al.* (1975)	Simplification	27	40	<0.05
Ley *et al.* (1973)	Explicit categorisation	50	64	<0.05
Reynolds *et al.* (1981)	Explicit categorisation			
	5 days	48	66	n.s.
	6 weeks	55	64	n.s.
Kupst *et al.* (1975)	Repetition: by physician	76	90	<0.05
	by patient		91	<0.05
Bertakis (1977)	Repetition by patient	62	83	<0.05
Bradshaw *et al.* (1975)	Use of specific			
	statements		16	51	<0.01
Ley *et al.* (1976b)	Mixture of Doctor: A	52	61	<0.05
	the above B	56	70	<0.05
	methods C	57	73	<0.05
	D	59	80	<0.05
Analogue studies				
Ley *et al.* (1973)	Explicit categorisation	43	61	<0.05
Ley (1979a)	Explicit categorisation	36	50	<0.05
Ley (1979a)	Repetition by presenter	33	47	<0.05

INCREASING PATIENTS' SATISFACTION BY INCREASING UNDERSTANDING AND RECALL

If patients' dissatisfaction with communications results in part from their not understanding and not recalling what they are told it should be possible to increase satisfaction by increasing understanding and recall. Ley (1976a) attempted to increase patients' understanding by arranging for an experimental group of medical inpatients to receive extra visits from a physician during which the physician tried to ensure that patients had understood what they had been told. Because extra attention of this sort might in itself increase satisfaction a placebo condition was used. In this condition patients also received extra visits from the physician, but the topics discussed were matters such as adjustment to hospital, problems caused by hospitalisation, and ways in which hospital stay could be improved for patients in general. In addition there was a 'no intervention' control group who received no extra visits. The results were as predicted: 80 per cent of the experimental group were satisfied with communications as compared with 52 per cent of the controls and 41 per cent of the placebo group.

Ley, Swinson, Bradshaw and Kincey (1974) attempted to replicate this finding with surgical inpatients. The attempt was not successful. The percentages of the experimental, control, and placebo groups who were satisfied with communications were 72, 75, and 84 per cent respectively. These percentages did not differ significantly from one another. However, even in this study there was a significant correlation between reported understanding and satisfaction with communications ($r = +0.45$, $p < 0.001$). The difference in results between the medical and surgical patients might well be due to the much higher levels of satisfaction with communications found in the surgical group as a whole.

Working in a family practice setting, Bertakis (1977), as has already been mentioned, made a successful attempt to increase recall by the use of repetition. However, not only did the experimental group recall more than the control group, but they were also more satisfied. It was also found that, within groups, satisfaction was related to amount recalled.

Thus there is at least some evidence that methods likely to increase understanding and recall lead to increases in patients' satisfaction, and there is further evidence supporting this

85

conclusion from studies of the use of written materials, e.g. George, Waters and Nicholas (1983).

EFFECTS OF IMPROVING MEMORY BY USE OF REMINDERS

Several researchers have shown that the use of telephoned or postal reminders can increase compliance. Most of this research has attempted to increase the probability that a patient will keep an appointment or attend for follow-up. Obviously the determinants of broken appointments involve many factors other than failures of memory. (For general reviews of this literature see Dunbar, Marshall and Hovell (1979), Deyo and Inui (1980) and Levy and Loftus (1983).) It is also true that reminders might well serve functions other than that of simple memory aids. For example, writing to or telephoning a patient about an appointment can convey the message that the clinic is a caring or efficient place, and this of course could affect patients' attitudes and behaviour in relation to it. Nevertheless it is probably fair to assume that, whatever other functions reminders serve, they will reduce forgetting of appointment times and details.

There appears to be a reasonably consistent increase in appointment keeping following a reminder, and it seems that mailed and phoned reminders are of about equal effectiveness. Thus Gates and Colborn (1976) compared three groups of patients, one of which received a telephone reminder, the second of which received a mailed reminder, and the third of which received no reminder. In the postal reminder group compliance was 84 per cent, in the telephoned group it was 80 per cent, and in the control group 55 per cent. These findings were echoed in a study by Shepard and Moseley (1976) in which 56 per cent of the group receiving the posted reminder attended for their appointment, as did 62 per cent of the telephoned group, and 43 per cent of the controls.

Other studies have investigated the effects of mailed reminders. Nazarian, Mechaber, Charney and Coulter (1974) reported that the use of a mailed reminder increased appointment keeping from 48 to 64 per cent. Similarly Meller and Anderson (1976) found appointment keeping to increase from 69 to 83 per cent when a mailed reminder was used. Further confirmation of the effectiveness of this strategy comes from

Levy and Claravell (1977) who reported that the group who received a mailed reminder kept 64 per cent of appointments as opposed to the 47 per cent of appointments kept by those not receiving a reminder. The effect of combining telephoned and postal reminders was investigated by Reiss and Bailey (1982), who found that the combined reminder led to 70 per cent of patients keeping their appointments as opposed to 38 per cent in the usual condition, where reminders were not issued. Frimon, Finney, Rapoff and Christophersen (1985) also used a combination of mailed and phoned reminders, and in addition provided a free parking permit to allow easier access to the clinic. This package led to 75 per cent of appointments being kept, compared with 56 per cent for the control group.

These studies are summarised in Table 6.3, where it can be seen that, on average, across a reasonably wide range of types of patient compliance in appointment keeping a further 20 per cent or so of patients keep their appointments when a reminder of some sort is used.

Table 6.3: Effects of reminders on compliance in appointment keeping

| Investigation | Patients ($n =$) | Percentage keeping appointment | | | | |
		Control	Postal	Phoned	Both	p
Nazarian et al. (1974)	Pediatric (670)	48	64	—	—	<0.001
Gates & Colborn (1976)	Primary care (227)	55	84	— 80	—	<0.05 <0.05
Mellor and Anderson (1976)	Pediatric (566)	69	83	—	—	<0.01
Shepard and Moseley (1976)	(a) Pediatric (932)	43	56 —	— 62	—	<0.05 <0.05
	(b) Pediatric without telephone (97)	33	50	—	—	<0.05
Levy and Claravell (1977)	Pediatric (98)	47	64	—	—	<0.05
Morse et al. (1981)	Pediatric (766)	62	64	—	—	n.s.
Reiss and Bailey (1982)	Dental (47)	38	—	—	70	<0.05
Frimon et al. (1985)	Pediatric	56	—	—	75	<0.01

In general there appears to be a relationship between the probability of a patient keeping an appointment and the time elapsing between the making of that appointment and the date when it is due to be kept (Deyo and Inui, 1980). Most of this evidence is derived from studies which have simply investigated the correlation between the time elapsing and the percentage of appointments kept. This methodology unfortunately makes for difficulties in interpretation of any association so found. For example perhaps patients who seem more concerned about their condition are given earlier appointments, and perhaps these are the patients most likely to keep their appointments anyway. Or perhaps patients who are keenest to attend are also those who are most persistent in requesting early appointments. These are quite plausible explanations of the association and of course there are other possible explanations as well. What is needed to settle the matter is evidence from experiments where patients are assigned in some random manner to varying lengths of delay.

Two such experiments have been reported by Bauman, Reiss and Bailey (1984), who found in both that greater delay led to more broken appointments. In the first of these experiments people wishing to attend a family planning clinic were assigned to a one-week or to a three-week wait before their appointment. Of those who had to wait one week 75 per cent kept their appointment, but only 57 per cent of those who had to wait three weeks did so. The second experiment involved patients attending for gynaecological screening. These patients were assigned to either an appointment on the following day or to an appointment two weeks later. A total of 72 per cent of the first group kept their appointments as opposed to 52 per cent of the second group. Thus the results of these experimental studies support the suggestion of the correlational investigations in finding an association between delay in appointment and frequency of broken appointments.

In view of these findings it is particularly interesting to note that it seems as though the effects of reminders are at their strongest in precisely those situations where there is a long delay before the appointment date. In the study by Nazarian *et al.* (1974) it was found that, without reminders, 50–56 per cent of patients kept their appointments when the appointment was made 12–28 days ahead, 33 per cent when it was 29–35 days ahead, and 43 per cent when it was more than 35 days ahead.

Corresponding percentages for those receiving reminders were 62–71, 55 and 68 per cent respectively. It can be seen that there is a greater increase in appointments kept when reminders are used when the delay is longer. This finding is supported by the investigation of Levy and Claravell (1977) in which it was found that without reminders 54 per cent of patients whose appointment was made 14 or fewer days in advance kept their appointments, while only 38 per cent whose appointments were made 15 or more days in advance kept them. However, when patients received reminders these percentages rose to 60 and 68 per cent respectively. It seems, therefore, that reminders are particularly effective in overcoming the decline in appointment keeping attributable to increasing interval between the date when an appointment is made and its due date.

We can therefore conclude that postal and telephone reminders are a reliable way of decreasing patients' non-compliance in appointment keeping. On average it can be expected that an extra 20 per cent of patients will keep their appointments if reminders are issued. Further, reminders might be particularly useful in reducing appointment breaking in those situations where it is especially likely to occur because of delay between the making of the appointment and the date when it is due to be kept.

The only slight worry in accepting this conclusion arises from the investigation by Morse, Coulter, Nazarian, and Napodano (1981) in which was studied the effect of *not* issuing a postal reminder to patients attending a clinic where, following their successful use in the investigation of Nazarian *et al.* (1974), the issue of such reminders had become routine. While in the earlier study providing mailed reminders had increased the rate of keeping appointments from 48 to 64 per cent, in the later study *not* mailing a reminder had no effect on appointment keeping. Among those who received reminders 64 per cent of appointments were kept, compared with 62 per cent amongst those not receiving reminders.

THE USE OF 'MECHANICAL' AIDS TO MEMORY

Attempts have been made to reduce patients' non-compliance by the provision of packs, stickers, or other devices likely to reduce their forgetting about when to take their medicine. These devices have included the following:

(a) auditory signals;
(b) tear-off calendars with each day's dose(s) and times of taking;
(c) tablet identification cards with the schedule for each dose placed alongside an example of the pill to which it refers;
(d) pill wheels and other weekly packs which have a compartment for each day of the week, each of which in turn can hold a number of doses, usually four;
(e) packs which have the tablets arranged by time of day as well as day of the week, thus all of the tablets to be taken at breakfast on Wednesday will be together in a group marked 'Breakfast, Wednesday';
(f) reminder stickers for placing near points where they are likely to be seen when it is time to take the tablet;
(g) colour-coded bottles, colours corresponding to different times of day.

Azrin and Powell (1969) devised a pill container which emitted an auditory signal at the time the medication should be taken. The signal could be switched off by turning a knob, which also controlled a mechanism for ejecting a pill into the patient's hand. The duration of the signal was one minute. In an analogue study it was found that mean errors made by subjects with this device were the same as those for subjects with an ordinary pill container.

In an investigation of elderly patients MacDonald, Mac-Donald and Phoenix (1977) compared three groups. These were a control group, a group who received counselling about their medication, and a group who received counselling plus one of three memory aids. The memory aids were a pill wheel, a tear-off calendar, and a tablet identification card. Data were provided in the report of this research which allow calculation of the percentage of patients taking too many or two few tablets. As these are the errors which would be expected to be affected by the memory aids, they have been used in this review. The original paper uses a wider definition of medication errors, hence the figures given here differ a little from the original. A final complication is that the appropriate control group against which to assess the effects of the memory is the group who received counselling alone. In the group receiving the memory aids 42 per cent were judged compliant compared with 57 per cent compliant in the control group. The difference is not statistically significant. This result has to be interpreted with some caution as the pill wheel was too difficult for many of these elderly patients to cope with. Its use was physically beyond them.

Wandless and Davie (1977) also assessed the effectiveness of a tear-off calendar and a tablet identification card. Elderly patients were assigned either to a group receiving a calendar, or to a group receiving a chart, or to a control group who received neither memory aid. Both the calendar and the card were effective in reducing medication errors, and they did not differ significantly from one another in effectiveness.

The effectiveness of a compartmentalised box, the Dosett, was studied by Crome, Akehurst and Keet (1980). Elderly patients who received their medication in this special container made about the same number of medication errors as those who received the ordinary container. However, Rehder, McCoy, Blackwell, Whitehead, and Robinson (1980) found that the use of a dosett container significantly increased the percentage of patients who took 95 per cent or more of the prescribed medication, although it had no effect on average medication errors. Also of interest in this study was the finding that of those who could still be contacted six months later 54 per cent said they were still using the device.

Spriet, Beiler, Dechorgnat and Simon (1980) assigned elderly patients at random to receiving reminder stickers or to a control condition. The stickers were to be placed in situations where they would be likely to be seen at medicine taking times, and thus remind the patient. This intervention was ineffective in increasing compliance.

Crome, Curl, Boswell, Corless and Lewis (1982) assessed the effectiveness of a new calendar pack which they called the 'C-Pak'. This was a device which packaged pills in terms of the day of the week on which they should be taken and the time of day at which they should be taken. Elderly patients were assigned to either the 'C-Pak' or a control group. Medication errors were virtually the same in both groups.

Colour coding was used by Martin and Mead (1982) in an attempt to reduce medication errors in elderly patients. The colour codes referred to time of day. Thus morning was coded red; lunchtime, yellow; evening, blue; and night/suppertime, black. A 28-compartment tray, also colour coded, was used as an additional aid. Patients were randomly assigned to receiving either colour-coded bottles, or colour-coded bottles and the colour-coded tray, or to a control group, who received ordinary bottles. Colour coding the bottles had no effect on medication errors, but the combination of colour-coded bottles and tray greatly reduced errors.

Overall, this variety of ingenious ideas to improve memory has had somewhat disappointing results. These are summarised in Table 6.4.

Table 6.4: Effectiveness of mechanical memory aids in reducing non-compliance

Investigation	Memory aid	Mean percentage medication error		p
		Control	Aided	
Azrin and Powell (1969)	Auditory signal	16	11	n.s.
Wandless and Davie	Tear-off calendar	28	18	<0.01
(1977)	Tablet chart		21	<0.01
Crome *et al.* (1980)	Dosett box	8.5	6.2	n.s.
Crome *et al.* (1982)	'C-Pak'	26.1	26.2	n.s.
Martin and Mead	Colour-coded bottles	17.1	17.3	n.s.
(1982)	As above plus tray		1.7	<0.01
		Percentage compliant		
MacDonald *et al.*	Pill wheel, tear-off	57	42	n.s.
(1977)	calendar, or tablet card			
Rehder *et al.* (1980)	Dosett box	54[a]	90[a]	<0.01
Spriet *et al.* (1980)	Reminder stickers	61	63	n.s.

Note: [a]estimated from histogram

SUMMARY

The results reviewed in this chapter can be summarised as follows.

   (a) Recall of the content of orally presented communications
       can be increased by the use of:
       (1) primacy effects;
       (2) stressing the importance of particular content.
   (b) The amount recalled can be increased by the use of:
       (1) simplification;
       (2) explicit categorisation;
       (3) repetition;

(4) use of specific rather than general statements;
(5) mixtures of the above.

(c) Telephoned and mailed reminders are effective in reducing the frequency with which appointments are broken.

(d) A variety of mechanical aids to memory have been tried, mainly with elderly patients and mainly without success.

(e) Data from one study, (Rehder *et al.*, 1980), suggests that in the long term, patients' non-compliance in using the mechanical devices with which they have been issued, will be found to be at the level of non-compliance in general.

One effective method for increasing patients' recall and knowledge which has not been discussed in this chapter is the use of written supplementary information. Evidence about its effectiveness will be reviewed in Chapter 8.

7

Another Problem: Non-compliance by Health Care Professionals

INTRODUCTION

Even if it were possible to produce a set of guidelines and procedures leading to significant improvement in communication it is most unlikely that all health care professionals would use them. This is because, as we shall see, professionals are just as likely to be non-compliant with advice and rules for the provision of the best health care as their patients are in adhering to the advice given to them.

The problem of non-compliance by professionals has received much less attention than that devoted to non-compliance by patients. Gordis (1979) made some reference to the problem, and Ley (1981) provided a brief review of studies in the area. All health professions have explicit and implicit guidelines for what is proper and adequate care, and it is deviation from these that will be labelled as professional non-compliance. In what follows it will emerge that members of a wide variety of health care professions are frequently found to be non-compliant in this sense. It is probably legitimate to assume that professions not mentioned in this chapter are equally non-compliant, but have had the good fortune not to have had this aspect of their behaviour studied and published.

THE MAGNITUDE OF THE PROBLEM

Because the writer is a psychologist it is probably only fair to start this review with some data on psychologists' non-compliance. Psychologists often administer intelligence tests to children, and the information so obtained is often used to make important decisions about a child's future. To be useful intelligence tests have to have strictly standardised rules for their administration and scoring. It is true that some will argue that there will be occasions when, on clinicial grounds these procedures have to be modified, but even they accept that in the vast bulk of cases the test must be administered and scored in the prescribed manner. Miller, Chansky, and Gredler (1970) gave 32 trainees a completed test protocol to score. (The test was the Wechsler Intelligence Scale for Children.) Thirty made errors in scoring, and these trainees gave IQs ranging from 76 to 93 to the same protocol. A further study by Miller and Chansky (1972), again using Wechsler's test, showed that such errors were not restricted to trainees. In this investigation Miller and Chansky selected at random 200 names from the American Psychological Association's lists of those who were either Fellows or Members of the School or Clinical Psychology Divisions. Each was sent a test protocol and asked to score it. Of the 64 psychologists who complied with this request 54 made scoring errors. These resulted in IQs ranging from 78 to 95 being awarded to the protocol.

Several researches have investigated the compliance of pharmacists in the USA, most of which have involved sending pseudo-patients into pharmacies to get a prescription filled, or to purchase a medicine or drug. These pseudo-patients are of course accomplices of the experimenter, who normally go through a prepared routine to assess and observe the health-care professional's behaviour in situations of interest.

Knapp, Wolf, Knapp and Rudy (1969) reported two studies which used this method. In the first of these a pseudo-patient visited 36 pharmacies, and established in casual conversation that he was a diabetic. He then tried to purchase and asked for information about a decongestant medicine. The decongestant requested was one which was likely to have severe effects on the control of blood sugar levels in diabetics. Despite this, in 30 out of the 36 pharmacies the medicine was provided without any comment about its potential danger to diabetics.

In the second study, a pseudo-patient visited 12 pharmacies to present a prescription for a monoamine oxidase inhibitor. The same person had, one week previously, visited each pharmacy with a prescription for imipramine. If these two drugs are taken concurrently there can be lethal adverse reactions.

Despite rules about keeping records and checking on patients, only one of the pharmacies noted the dangerous combination of drugs. Further, there can be dangerous interactions between monoamine oxidase inhibitors and common foodstuffs, e.g. cheese, spinach, hence it is considered good practice to warn patients about these. In only one of the pharmacies did this happen.

Wertheimer, Schefter and Cooper (1973) also used the pseudo-patient technique in two studies. In the first the accomplice visited pharmacies to purchase an anti-diarrhoeal for an 18 month-old infant. The age of the patient was conveyed to the pharmacist. Despite the fact that the medicine requested was clearly labelled as being unsuitable for use with children under three years of age, except under medical direction, in only 18 out of 50 pharmacies was the purchaser advised to consult a doctor. In their second study, these investigators checked on pharmacists' willingness to sell quinine to a 17 year old, and whether any sold was labelled in such a way as to meet statutory requirements. In the USA quinine is used to 'cut' heroin. Four out of 30 pharmacies refused to sell heroin to the youth. Of the 27 which did agree to sell it only one labelled it in such a way as to meet legal requirements.

In addition to investigating the adequacy of advice about the medication provided, Rowles, Keller and Gavin (1974) assessed the accuracy with which the medicine was made up. The study involved 100 pharmacies, to which a pseudo-patient took a prescription. In only 20 were adequate directions for use given, and in only 28 were the ingredients accurate to within plus or minus 5 per cent. Only five out of the 100 pharmacies were adequate in both respects.

In an investigation in Washington State, Campbell and Grisafe (1975) studied pharmacists' compliance with state regulations about informing patients about medication. Of 200 pharmacies, chosen by random sampling procedures and visited by a pseudo-patient only 94 were found to provide adequate oral instructions and in only 18 were warnings given that the prescribed drug would interact adversely with aspirin.

Morris, Myers, Gibbs and Lao (1980) conducted research to see whether pharmacists were complying with regulations that they should issue a patient package insert when providing customers with oestrogens. Pharmacies were selected by a stratified random sampling technique to cover 20 cities in the USA.

This time the pseudo-patients were members of the US Food and Drug Administration's field staff, and they visited 271 pharmacies. At each a prescription for an oestrogen product was presented and made up. Despite regulations requiring the issuing of a leaflet with such products, this was provided spontaneously by only 39 per cent of the pharmacies. A further 55 per cent provided the leaflet when the observer requested one, but the regulation was intended to see that this happened spontaneously.

An investigation into nurses' non-compliance with procedures for issuing medicines was conducted by Hofling, Brotzman, Dalrymple, Graves and Pierce (1966). The hospitals in which the nurses worked, and in which the experiment took place, had rules about the administering of medicines to patients. In essence these stated that a nurse should not administer a new medicine to a patient unless a doctor known to the nurse requested, in writing, that a drug on the ward stocklist be administered. In the experiment (a) the drug was not on the ward stock list, (b) the doctor making the request was unknown to the nurse and, (c) the request that the patient be given the drug was made by telephone. If this were not enough, on the package of the drug requested it was clearly and visibly stated that the maximum daily dose was 10 mg. The dose that the nurse was asked to administer was 20 mg. The situation so described was put to groups of nurses, who were asked, if faced with it, what would they do: 94 per cent stated that they would not administer the medication under the circumstances. However, this contrasted sharply with what happened when the sequence of events happened in reality. Of the 22 nurses who received the telephone call in the circumstances described, 21 were willing to administer the medicine, and had to be stopped, medicine cup in hand, at the patient's bedside. Thus in real life 95 per cent were prepared to ignore the rules about medication.

Another major problem in hospitals is that of nosocomial infections. These are defined as infections which develop during, or sometimes after hospital stay, which were not present or incubating before the patient was admitted to hospital. The inference is of course that the infections were caught as a result of hospitalisation. Raven and Haley (1982) reported that approximately five per cent of the 32 million or so patients hospitalised in the USA each year will acquire such an infection, and the consequential immediate hospitalisation cost is of the order of a billion dollars each year. To this should be added the costs of later outpatient treatment, and of dealing with complications. More important than these financial implications is the fact that in the USA an estimated 15 000 patients a year die from nosocomical infections, and obviously many others suffer as a consequence of them. Part of this problem is due to non-compliance with infection control procedures on the part of hospital personnel. These include such relatively simple things as proper handwashing, wearing masks in isolation rooms, and disposing of used syringes properly. Raven and Haley (1982) reported the results of a survey conducted with large samples of nurses to assess their likely compliance with infection control procedures in three hypothetical situations.

In the first of these, nurses were asked what they would do if a doctor requested that for psychological reasons a child should be moved out of isolation, even though the child still had a staphyloccocal infection which was still oozing pus. Sixty-one per cent of nurses said that they would not comply with this request.

In the second situation, a doctor needs to send a patients' urine sample to the laboratory immediately, and instructs the nurse to proceed with catheterisation, even though both doctor and nurse know that the nurse has accidentally contaminated the catheter. Seventy-eight per cent of nurses claimed that they would not comply with this request.

In the third situation a doctor asks the nurse to allow a child to keep a pet turtle in his room as a morale booster, even though hospital policy bans turtles because of the high risk of salmonella infection. This time 76 per cent of nurses claimed that they would not agree to this.

Some idea of how realistic these hypothetical situations were can be derived from data presented by Raven and Haley which show that 38 per cent of the nurses claimed that doctors make requests of this sort frequently or sometimes. In addition the nurses were asked how often they agreed to requests from doctors which infringed infection control policy. Eleven per cent said 'almost always'; 19 per cent said 'frequently'; 44 per cent said 'sometimes'; and 27 per cent said 'rarely or never'.

It should be noted of course that these are nurses' *statements* about what they would do. If the results of the study by Hofling *et al.* can be generalised it is likely that such reports will underestimate non-compliance with infection control rules.

The appropriateness with which medical practitioners prescribe antibiotics has also been the focus of a number of investigations. The criterion of appropriateness has been expert opinion. Gordis, Desi, and Schmerler (1976) investigated the use of antibiotics in cases of acute sore throat in children. The medical practitioners involved were either pediatricians or general physicians. It was found that 21 per cent of the former, and 76 per cent of the latter did not use these drugs appropriately, as assessed by the criterion of expert judgement.

Other studies of antibiotic use have reported their results in a different way. Instead of giving the percentage of professionals prescribing appropriately, they provide data on the percentage of patients receiving (a) an antibiotic when none was needed; or (b) the wrong antibiotic; or (c) the wrong dose. Scheckler and Bennett (1970), in a study of seven community hospitals, reported that 62 per cent of patients received an antibiotic when none was needed or received an inappropriate dose. A similar figure was arrived at by Roberts and Visconti (1972), who found, in a study of the patients of one hospital, that 66 per cent were receiving antibiotic treatment which was inappropriate in some way. Investigations at the University of Virginia Hospital (Kunin, Tupasi and Craig, 1973), and the Duke University Medical Centre (Castle, Wilfert, Cate, and Osterhout, 1977) also provided evidence of professional non-compliance in the proper use of antibiotics. The percentages of prescriptions, which were judged as not fitting the case were 51 per cent at Virginia, and 64 per cent at Duke. Kunin *et al.* also reported that, at Virginia, surgeons were more likely to be in error than physicians, with 58 per cent of the former and 39 per cent of the latter prescribing appropriately.

Findings such as these are not confined to the use of antibiotics. Avorn, Chen and Hartley (1982) studied prescribing habits of a random sample of physicians in the Boston (USA) area. The target drugs were cerebral vasodilators, and propoxythene. The first of these are not considered effective in the treatment of mental failure in the elderly. They are often prescribed for this group on the ground of the now discredited theory that dementia is due to restricted cerebral blood flow. Avorn *et al.* argue that the case against propoxythene is that in controlled trials it has not proved more effective than cheaper substitutes such as aspirin and codeine, and further that it has no other advantages over them. Thus they conclude that neither of these drugs can be prescribed appropriately. In their survey they found that 32 per cent of the sample used cerebral dilators for elderly confused patients, and that 41 per cent 'often', and 43 per cent 'occasionally' prescribed propoxythene. With a sample drawn from four states, a later study by Avorn and Sumerai (1983) also found evidence of widespread prescription of these drugs and of cephalosporins. The findings of this study are not reported in a way that lends itself to summary in terms of either physicians inappropriately prescribing, or patients improperly receiving these drugs.

The medical justification for injections given to patients by New Mexico medical practitioners was investigated by Brook and Williams (1975). During the period of the study over 95 000 injections were administered. It was found that 29 per cent of these could not be justified on medical grounds.

Cohen, Berner and Dubach (1985) investigated physicians' compliance with the guidelines of the Swiss Society against High Blood Pressure. In a two-month period the investigators discovered 151 patients with blood pressures high enough for them to need to be called back for a further check. Only 43 per cent were followed up in this way. Of these, 51 per cent were diagnosed as having hypertension and being in need of treatment. Of the patients in whom this need for treatment was established only 46 per cent received adequate treatment.

The frequency with which physicians conducted appropriate preventive investigations was investigated by Tierney, Hui and McDonald (1986). Test involved included tests for occult faecal blood and mammography. Only 10–15 per cent of the physicians conducted these tests in conditions where they were appropriate.

Nor does it seem that medical practitioners are very compliant with the advice that they should see that their patients are properly informed about their medication. Svarstadt (1974), and Webb (1976) reported investigations in which a qualified observer sat in on a series of consultations and assessed whether patients received adequate information from their doctors about the medicines prescribed for them. Svarstadt reported that a third of patients received such information, but Webb found that in her study, no patient received adequate information. Cockburn, Reid and Sanson-Fisher (1987), in a study involving recordings of 261 general practice consultations, in which an antibiotic was prescribed, found that the percentage of patients *not* receiving adequate information about various aspects of their treatment ranged from 25 to 100 per cent. Although 75 per cent were told that the medication was an antibiotic, fewer than 50 per cent were given any information about what sort of antibiotic it was, what side-effects might occur, for how long the drugs should be taken, what to do if a dose was missed and so on.

Finally with regard to non-compliance by medical practitioners, it has been for some time a strong recommendation of professional organisations that their members should regularly attend refresher courses. Cartwright (1967) reported that 44 per cent of British general practitioners did not do so.

The frequency with which dentists fail adequately to shield their patients when taking X-rays has also been investigated. The target behaviour has been the dentist's providing the patient with a lead apron to serve as a gonadal shield against secondary radiation. The American Dental Association and nearly every other pertinent organisation recommend that patients be provided with such shielding during X-ray. Unfortunately it looks as though this recommendation is one with which dentists do not always comply. Laws (1974) reported that over 90 per cent of dental X-rays were carried out without shielding. This finding received support from the study by Greene and Neistat (1983) who found, in a student sample who had recently had a dental X-ray, that 92 per cent had not been shielded. They further found that in half of a sample of 16 dental practices shielding was provided on less than 75 per cent of occasions, and that, in those practices, an average of 66 per cent of patients did not receive shielding. This figure was later confirmed in a pseudo-patient investigation. Student observers went as patients to these dental practices and it was found that only 31 per cent of them were provided with shielding. Fortunately, the experimenters had provided them with inconspicuous, but effective, gonadal shields, which they wore under their clothing.

Finally, Deliere and Schneider (1980) and Seaman, Greene and Watson-Perczel (1986) have reported on the accuracy with which emergency medical technicians carried out cardiopulmonary resuscitation techniques and found that between 39 and 79 per cent did not carry these out properly.

The results of these studies are summarised in Table 7.1.

This review has demonstrated that non-compliance is not

Table 7.1: Non-compliance by health care professionals with rules for good patient care

Investigation	Topic		Non-compliance
(a) Studies of percentage of professionals not complying			*% not complying*
1. Psychologists			
Miller *et al.* (1970)	Correct scoring of psychological tests		94
Miller and Chansky (1972)	Correct scoring of psychological tests		84
2. Pharmacists			
Knapp *et al.* (1969)	Warning of potentially dangerous drug interaction or drug danger	(a)	83
		(b)	92
Wertheimer *et al.* (1973)			64
Campbell and Grisafe (1975)	Adequate labelling and counselling about medicine use		91
Wertheimer *et al.* (1973)			81
Rowles *et al.* (1974)			80
Campbell and Grisafe (1975)			53
Morris *et al.* (1980)	Issuing oestrogen patient package insert		61
3. Nurses			
Hofling *et al.* (1966)	Observing rules about medicine issue		95
Raven and Haley (1982)	Adhering to infection control procedures	(a)	39
		(b)	22
		(c)	24
4. Medical practitioners			
Cartwright (1967)	Attending refresher courses		44
Gordis *et al.* (1976)	Appropriate antibiotic prescribing	(a)	21
		(b)	76
		(c)	12
		(d)	59
5. Dentists			
Greene and Neistat (1983)	Shielding of patients during X-ray		50
6. Emergency medical technicians			
Deliere and Schneider (1980)	Correct performance of cardiopulmonary resuscitation Time since training:		
	(a) within 6 months		39
	(b) up to 12 months		47
	(c) more than 12 months		79
(b) Percentage of patients not receiving adequate care			*% not receiving*
1. Medical practitioners			
Scheckler and Bennett (1970)	Appropriate antibiotic therapy		62
Roberts and Visconti (1972)	Appropriate antibiotic therapy		66
Kunin *et al.* (1973)	Appropriate antibiotic therapy		51
Castle *et al.* (1977)	Appropriate antibiotic therapy		64
Svarstad (1974)	Adequate information about medication		66

Webb (1976)	Adequate information about medication		100
Cockburn *et al.* (1987)	Adequate information about medication		25–100
Brook and Williams (1975)	Appropriate injections		28
Avorn *et al.* (1982)	(a) Use of cerebral vasodilators		32
	(b) Use of unjustified analgesics		84
Cohen *et al.* (1985)	Follow-up of hypertensives		53
	Adequate treatment of hypertensives		54
Tierney *et al.* (1986)	Appropriate preventive care		85–90
2. Dentists			
Laws (1974)	Shielding during X-ray		90
Greene and Neistat (1983)	Shielding during X-ray	(a)	92
		(b)	66
		(c)	69

confined to patients. It can be argued therefore that it would perhaps be over-sanguine to expect that guidelines for improving communication will always be followed.

CAUSES OF NON-COMPLIANCE BY HEALTH-CARE PROFESSIONALS

It is likely that professional non-compliance is of two major types. On some occasions it is unintentional and due to lack of knowledge or forgetting of the rules and guidelines, or, in the case of sub-optimal prescribing of drugs, lack of familiarity with the literature on the current state of knowledge of the medication prescribed. In other cases it is intentional non-compliance and due to the beliefs and attitudes of the professional concerned, or to social pressures.

Examples of a relationship between the professional's knowledge and adherence to the best standard of care for patients can be found in the investigations by Watkins and Norwood (1978), Weaver, Ramirez, Dorfman and Raizner (1979) and Avorn *et al.* (1982). Watkins and Norwood reported a correlation of +0.47 between 55 pharmacists' knowledge of three medications and the adequacy of the counselling they gave to their patients about them. Adequacy of counselling behaviour was assessed by pseudo-patients, and knowledge by a true/false test. Using a knowledge test and a practical performance test, Weaver *et al.* found a correlation of +0.61 between retention of knowledge about resuscitation techniques and the skill with which they were performed. Avorn *et al.* also provided evidence of lack of knowledge in a sample of physicians. It was found that 71 per cent wrongly thought that impaired cerebral blood flow was a significant cause of senile dementia, with a further 15 per cent not sure whether this was true or not. In the case of propoxythene 49 per cent wrongly thought it to be more effective than aspirin. It will be recalled that in this sample of physicians about a third prescribed vasodilators for dementia, and 84 per cent prescribed propoxythene for pain. Avorn *et al.* suggest that these erroneous beliefs must come from advertising and conversation with drug company representatives, as they are clearly not in line with findings in the scientific literature. Most of the physicians seemed unaware of the influence of drug advertisements on their prescribing behaviour. Indeed, only two per cent thought that these had any influence on them. As the scientific literature does not seem to be an effective way of keeping physicians up to date, Avorn and his collaborators have explored the possibility of using 'unadvertisements', with results which will be discussed below.

Morris *et al.* (1980) tried to ascertain the reasons why the 61 per cent of pharmacists who did not spontaneously issue the oestrogen leaflet, as was required by the regulations, had failed to do so. Twenty-six per cent of the pharmacists stated that they had quite simply forgotten, and 7 per cent believed that it was to be issued at the request of the patient. It is also tempting to attribute the relationship between time since training and the decline in the percentage of emergency medical technicians and others correctly using cardiopulmonary resuscitation techniques reported by Weaver *et al.* (1979), Deliere and Schneider (1960), and Gass and Curry (1983) to forgetting. This decline in practical performance is accompanied by reductions in scores on tests of knowledge. Thus Weaver *et al.* reported that mean percentage correct answers on a test of knowledge of the techniques dropped from 87 to 76 per cent over a six month period. Similarly, Gass and Curry found that the mean knowledge scores of physicians dropped from 91 to 78 per cent over a twelve month period, while those for nurses dropped from 84 to 77.

Job satisfaction may also play some part in professionals' non-compliance. Thus Cartwright (1967) reported that general practitioners' attendance at refresher courses was associated with their level of job satisfaction. The higher this was, the more likely was the practitioner to attend refresher courses. Melville

(1979) investigated general practitioners' prescribing of drugs which were either inappropriate or against the use of which some official warning had been issued. These were: (a) practolol; (b) monoamine oxidase inhibitors; (c) anti-infective agents acting locally on the gut; (d) low doses of major tranquillisers for mild psychiatric problems in the elderly; (e) barbiturates; and, (f) amphetamine-like compounds. Melville found that doctors who continued to prescribe these drugs tended to have lower levels of job satisfaction than those who heeded the warnings against their use. In the case of the first four of these drugs job satisfaction was negatively correlated with their prescription.

Attitudinal factors are also probably of importance in professional non-compliance. For example, in their investigation of dentists' use of shields for their patients when X-rays were being used, Greene and Neistat (1983) found that dentists, who did not provide shielding, were as likely to be aware of the advice that they should, as dentists who complied with this advice. However, dentists who were non-compliant regarded shielding as being of less importance than the dentists who complied.

In the case of the non-compliance by nurses reported by Hofling *et al.* (1966), and Raven and Haley (1982) it is obvious that in many if not all cases the nurses knew that they were infringing regulations. For example, it will be recalled that 95 per cent of nurses who had the situation described to them by Hofling *et al.* stated that they would not infringe regulations in this way. Similarly it is clear from nurses' replies in the study by Raven and Haley that they were quite aware of what they should be doing, even if they did not do it. In these cases it is likely that at least part of the reason for non-compliance are the social pressures on nurses to comply with requests from doctors.

It is possible to argue that doctors themselves are often under social pressure from their patients, and that this is in some cases a contributing factor in sub-optimal prescribing. Although medical practitioners typically deny that they are influenced in this way (Melville, 1979: Avorn *et al.*, 1982), it seems that at least on some occasions patient influences are potent. Thus in the investigation by Avorn *et al.* 84 per cent of the physicians involved said that they 'often' or 'sometimes' prescribed a propoxythene analgesic 'because patients are not satisfied with an over-the-counter like aspirin'.

Thus, perhaps not surprisingly it looks as though poor knowledge, forgetting, beliefs, and social pressures contribute to non-compliance on the part of professionals. It is also interesting that a satisfaction variable should be of importance in this area as well as in patients' non-compliance.

THE REDUCTION OF PROFESSIONALS' NON-COMPLIANCE

An obvious strategy to use to decrease non-compliance by health-care professionals is to increase their knowledge. An educational intervention and the provision of a checklist was used by Brook and Williams (1975) in an attempt to reduce the frequency with which medically unjustifiable injections were administered. The intervention had a major impact on the overall use of injections which declined by 60 per cent. Unfortunately at the end of the study period the percentage of injections considered inappropriate on medical grounds was 40 per cent.

An increase in the quality of care and treatment of patients suffering from acute pharyngitis was obtained by the provision of guidelines by Grimm, Shimoni, Harlan and Estes (1975). Highly significant increases occurred for seven out of eight desirable physician behaviours. For example noting whether or not the patient had a history of rheumatic fever increased from 5 to 98 per cent.

Avorn and Sumerai (1983) attempted to increase physician knowledge by providing either written materials alone, or written materials plus face to face education informing the physician about the target drugs, which were cephalexin, propoxythene, and papaverine. The written information, which was sent to the physicians at regular intervals, consisted of (a) booklets very similar to publications like the *FDA Drug Bulletin* or *Prescribers Journal,* and (b) a series of 'unadvertisements', in which the same information was presented in a four colour, profusely illustrated, visually appealing format. The group receiving written materials alone was further divided into those who received only the booklets and those who received booklets and 'unadvertisements'. Physicians assigned to this last condition also received information pamphlets for distribution to patients. The face to face group in addition to receiving all of the written materials, were visited twice in the experimental period by pharmaceutical educators. At these visits the educators reviewed the information contained in the written materials, and tried to encourage the physicians to move in the direction of reduced use of the target drugs. Four hundred and thirty-five physicians were randomly assigned to one of these groups or to a control group who received no intervention. The results showed that the use of written materials alone was ineffective in changing prescribing behaviour, but that the face to face condition successfully reduced prescribing of all three target drugs. Further, this effect was still present nine months after the start of the face to face intervention and was showing no sign of diminishing.

Unfortunately face to face educational attempts to improve treatment of hypertensive patients were found not to be successful by Cohen *et al.* (1985). Physicians who had not been complying with guidelines for the treatment of hypertension were given feedback about their performance, reminded of the guidelines, and reminded of the details of the US Veterans Administration's and the Australian Intervention Group's results concerning the treatment of hypertension. This intervention had no effect on either the proportion of patients asked by the physicians to attend for follow-up, nor on the proportion receiving adequate treatment. A second intervention, which was successful, involved arranging for nurses routinely to make a second appointment for any patient falling within the guidelines, and attaching a highly visible sticker to the patient's casenotes. Under these conditions 83 per cent of patients were followed up, and of those in this group who required treatment, 77 per cent received it.

Computer-based prompts and reminders have also been used to increase quality of care. De Dombal, Leaper, Horrocks, Staniland and McCann (1974) reported on the effectiveness of computer-aided diagnosis in cases of abdominal pain. The proportion of appendices which perforated before surgery fell from 36 per cent to 4 per cent while the system was in use. Similarly, the negative laparotomy rate dropped from about 25 per cent to 7 per cent. Unfortunately, when the use of the computer aid ceased both of these rates returned to near their previous levels.

McDonald (1977), McDonald, Murray, Jeris, Bharvaga, Seeger and Blevins (1977), and MacDonald (1979) described a computer system which recorded patient details during diagnosis and treatment. Inevitably during these processes findings are made to which the physician might need to respond. For example given certain features of the patient's history and current laboratory findings there might be a case for using one drug rather than another. The computer program described by MacDonald and colleagues is arranged to alert the physician to this sort of situation and make suggestions about changes in drug regimen, further investigations, and so on. MacDonald (1979) reported the results of two studies. In the first of these conducted in a diabetes clinic, physicians responded to 36 per cent of drug-related events when the computer was available, compared with 11 per cent in the control condition when it was not. The second study, which was conducted in a general medical clinic, reported similar findings. The targets of the study were the use of medications and the tests used to monitor their effectiveness and toxicity. The physicians involved responded to 22 per cent of events in the control condition, and to 51 per cent in the computer condition. These results suggest that the provision of reminders to physicians can improve clinical performance. Further studies by this group have confirmed the usefulness of both computer reminders at the time of consultation and monthly feedback of performance based on computer records in improving physician performance, e.g. McDonald, Hui, Smith, Tierney, Cohen, Weinberger and McCabe (1984), Tierney, Hui and McDonald (1986).

Behavioural methods have also been used to decrease professionals' non-compliance. In order to increase dentists' provision of X-ray shielding for their patients Greene and Neistat (1983) used feedback and prompting. Dentists who were not providing shielding received a package pointing out that they were (a) not providing shielding; (b) reminding them of the official view that shielding should be provided; (c) presenting them with data about how frequently their patients and those of other local dentists were given this protection, (d) informing them that there would be further monitoring of this problem; and (e) stickers to attach to the X-ray machine and its switch containing the instruction: 'Use lead apron'. In addition a further letter was sent. Following this intervention virtually all patients received shielding, and this was maintained for the follow-up period of a year or so. Seaman *et al.* (1986) also reported success in the use of behavioural methods in the training and maintenance of the correct use of cardiopulmonary resuscitation techniques.

As we shall see, there are similarities between these methods successful in reducing non-compliance in professionals and those which have proved successful in reducing non-compliance in patients.

SUMMARY

The findings reviewed above can be summarised as follows:

(a) Non-compliance by health-care professionals seems to be surprisingly common.
(b) Factors involved in this non-compliance include: lack of knowledge, failures of memory, low job satisfaction, and susceptibility to social pressures.
(c) There is some preliminary evidence that educational efforts, reminders, and behavioural strategies can sometimes reduce such non-compliance.

While professionals' non-compliance is obviously of interest in its own right, in the present context it is the implication that guidelines for improving communication are likely to be frequently ignored which is of most interest. Even if it could be shown that modifying the clinicians' communicative behaviour in certain ways reliably led to better informed patients, better compliance, and improved outcomes, it would be unrealistic to expect that there would not be a substantial proportion of clinicians who would be unaffected by these findings. This obviously raises the question of what alternative or supplementary techniques might be employed to successfully communicate information to patients. An obvious possibility to consider is the use of written information.

8

The Use of Written Information for Patients

INTRODUCTION

Given that oral communications often fail in that they are frequently not understood and frequently forgotten, and the further complications produced by the non-compliance of health-care professionals, it is obviously tempting to consider the use of written information as a way of supplementing and improving communications. In theory written information has a number of advantages. It can be constructed in such a way as to enhance both understanding and memory. The content can be written so as to ensure coverage of all important points, and it also provides a permanent record of the information. This of course means that it is available for later consultation should the need arise. A further advantage is that people appear to be favourably disposed towards written informtion about health matters. For example, it is clear from survey evidence that people in general desire to have written information about medication. Morris and Groft (1982) reviewed a number of US studies of this topic and found the median percentage wishing for written information about their medication was 77 per cent.

Further, the majority of patients receiving written information express favourable attitudes towards it. For example the major study conducted by the Rand Corporation for the US Food and Drug Administration, Kanouse, Berry, Hayes-Roth, Rogers and Winkler (1981a) found that in answer to various questions 75–93 per cent of those receiving leaflets about erythromycin, 58–90 per cent of those receiving a leaflet about flurazepam, and 27–84 per cent of those receiving a leaflet about oral contraceptives expressed favourable attitudes towards the usefulness of the leaflets. Other studies report similar findings (Fleckenstein, Joubert, Lawrence, Patsner, Mazullo and Lasagna, 1976; Hladik and White, 1976; Mazis, Morris and Gordon, 1978; Weibert, 1977; Dwyer and Hammel, 1978; Romankiewicz, Gotz and Carlin, 1978; Udkow, Lasagna, Weintraub and Tamoshunas, 1979; Gauld, 1981; George, Waters and Nicholas, 1983). This last study also found that patients who received written information were more satisfied with their treatment as a whole. Further, there are some suggestions that larger amounts of information are preferred to lesser amounts (Morris, Mazis and Gordon, 1977; Mazis, Morris and Gordon, 1978; Morris and Kanouse, 1980). Written information is therefore likely to be welcomed by most of its recipients.

This chapter will examine the overall effectiveness of written information, and discuss some of the problems associated with its use. In brief it will be argued that to be effective written information has to be noticed, read, understood, believed, and remembered. As will be seen these conditions do not always obtain.

In what follows frequent reference will be made to the study (already mentioned above) of written information for patients, about drugs prescribed for them, conducted for the US Food and Drug Administration by the Rand Corporation. Among the reports arising from this research are those of Berry, Kanouse, Hayes-Roth, Rogers, Winkler, and Garfinkle (1981), in which the drug concerned was flurazepam; Kanouse, Berry, Hayes-Roth, Rogers, Winkler, and Garfinkle (1981), in which the drug concerned was oestrogen; and Winkler, Kanouse, Berry, Hayes-Roth, Rogers, and Garfinkle (1981), in which the drug concerned was erythromycin.

Subjects, who were English speaking and aged 18 or over, were recruited for these studies with the cooperation of 69 pharmacies in the Los Angeles area. Eligible subjects were approached by the pharmacist, when presenting or collecting a prescription, and told that the pharmacist was involved in a study about the information people have about prescription drugs. The potential subjects were given a written description of what would be required of them if they agreed to cooperate. If the subject agreed to cooperate they signed a form indicating this, and were later interviewed by telephone. For those prescribed erythromycin this occurred at least 3 days, and for the others, at least 10 days after the prescription had been made

111

up. Note that no attempt was made to confine the study to new users, and that 67 per cent of the flurazepam users, 95 per cent of the oestrogen users and 41 per cent of the erythromycin patients had used the drug previously. Percentages of those eligible, agreeing at the pharmacy to cooperate, were 52 per cent for flurazepam, 51 per cent for oestrogen, and 60 per cent for erythromycin. Telephone interviews were completed with 87 per cent of those agreeing to cooperate. In the event interviews were conducted with 369 people taking flurazepam, 572 taking oestrogens, and 880 taking erythromycin.

This research investigated the effects on behavioural and attitudinal reactions to leaflets about these drugs of:

(a) specificity of instructions;
(b) amount of explanation given;
(c) highlighting information about the risks and dangers of using the drug;
(d) making the text easier to understand;
(e) presenting the text in outline as opposed to full sentences and paragraphs;
(f) total amount of information provided.

Findings of this large-scale project will be reviewed as appropriate in the following sections of this and the next chapters.

THE EFFECTIVENESS OF WRITTEN INFORMATION IN IMPROVING COMMUNICATION

Written information about medication has been evaluated in relation to its effectiveness in (a) increasing patients' knowledge, (b) increasing compliance, and (c) improving outcomes of treatment. Reviews of the research on this topic have been provided by Morris and Halperin (1979), Morris and Groft (1982), and Ley and Morris (1984). The findings of this research are summarised in Table 8.1, where it can be seen that in the majority of studies the provision of written information about medication has been found to have beneficial effects. The effects are most pronounced when the criterion is increased knowledge, less so when the criterion is increased compliance, and smallest of all when the criterion is demonstrated therapeutic benefit. Nevertheless this evidence suggests an overall

Table 8.1: The effects of the provision of written information about medication on knowledge, compliance, and outcome

Effect	Number of studies	Per cent showing effect
Increased knowledge	32	97
Increased compliance	25	60
Improved outcome	7	57

beneficial effect from the provision of written information about medication.

Written information can be effective in other clinical situations as well. For example, Ellis, Hopkin, Leitch and Crofton (1979) assigned 56 patients being discharged from an acute general medical and respiratory unit to two conditions. In both conditions patients were verbally given information about diagnosis, general advice, drug treatment, prognosis, and follow-up arrangements. In addition one group also received a copy of this information in writing. At follow up, the percentages of patients receiving written information who knew the diagnosis was 70 per cent; the general advice, 23 per cent; treatment, 93 per cent; and prognosis, 60 per cent. Corresponding percentages for those who received only the verbal communication were 31, 12, 55 and 46. These differences were significant for diagnosis, advice, and treatment, and this was despite the fact that the physicians involved thought that their verbal explanations were of great lucidity.

Working in a surgical context, Young and Humphrey (1985) reported that a group of women undergoing hysterectomy and who received a booklet about how to survive hospital and cope with anxiety, showed less postoperative pain and distress, and were discharged from hospital more quickly than controls who did not receive the booklet. Similarly, Wallace (1986) compared the effectiveness of two booklets in increasing knowledge and reducing anxiety in patients undergoing gynaecological surgery. It was found that one of the booklets was effective in reducing anxiety.

Further examples can be drawn from the treatment of obesity, where Ley (1986b), reviewing studies by Hagen (1974), Ley (1978), Stunkard (1979), Jeffery and Gerber (1982), and Pezzot-Pearce, LeBow and Pearce (1982), concluded that weight losses achieved by obese persons exposed to written information alone ranged from 3.4 to 7.4 kg over periods ranging from 8 to 16 weeks, and 4.5 to 7.4 kg over longer periods. These weight losses are not very different from those obtained by the groups in these studies who received much more personal attention.

Two final examples are the studies by Fisher, Scott Johnson, Porter, Bleich and Slack (1977), who found that a written communication was effective in increasing the purity of urine samples; and that of Fordham (1978), who found that written information led to cleaner colons in those attending for barium enema X-rays.

It is clear from this discussion that written information can often have beneficial effects in a wide range of clinically relevant contexts, but there is also evidence to show that these expected benefits do not always occur (Gatherer, Parfit, Porter, and Vessey, 1979). This raises the question of the conditions under which the provision of written information will and will not be effective. What problems are there in the effective use of written information?

IS WRITTEN INFORMATION READ BY ITS INTENDED AUDIENCE?

The answer to this question seems to be a qualified 'yes'. Table 8.2 summarises data available on the frequency with which people report having read leaflets and booklets given to them. By inference it can be assumed that these percentages represent minimum estimates of the percentages noticing the written materials. It can be seen that the frequency with which people report reading written health-related material provided for them ranges from 47 to 95 per cent.

These figures mean of course that in some cases substantial numbers of patients will not read literature given to them. If we examine the data reported by Berry *et al.*, Kabouse *et al.*, and Winkler *et al.* which were collected as parts of the same major study, and involved 32 separate samples of patients and three different medications, we find that there were no statistically significant differences in reported reading rates between leaflets for the three drugs, and that the overall mean percentage claiming to read the leaflets was 72 per cent, with a standard

Table 8.2: Frequency with which health-related materials are read

Investigation	Topic of information	Percentage claiming to have read the information provided
Brooks *et al.* (1964)	Baby care	58
Fleckenstein *et al.* (1976)	Oral contraceptive	91
Morris *et al.* (1977)	Oral contraceptive	94
Udkow *et al.* (1979)	Oestrogens	82
Visser (1980)	Hospitalisation and treatment	75
Cassileth *et al.* (1980)	Informed consent	
	(a) all patients	65
	(b) over-65s	47
Kanouse *et al.* (1981b)	Oestrogens (12 samples)	72
Berry *et al.* (1981)	Flurazepam (8 samples)	69
Winkler *et al.* (1981)	Erythromycin (12 samples)	74
Glasgow *et al.* (1981)	Smoking cessation	49–79
George *et al.* (1983)	(a) Penicillin	89
	(b) Anti-inflammatory drugs	95

deviation of approximately 9 per cent. It therefore seems reasonable to expect that just under three-quarters of patients will read leaflets about their medication. At present there are not enough data available to specify the conditions under which the figure will be higher or lower than this expectation.

MEASURING THE UNDERSTANDABILITY OF WRITTEN INFORMATION

The question of the understandability of written information has received a considerable amount of attention. The commonest method of evaluating these written materials has been to apply a readability formula, which yields an estimate of the reading grade required for understanding that material, and also permits an estimate to be made of the percentage of the population likely to understand the piece of writing. Currently there are well over 50 readability formulae available which are reviewed in detail by Klare (1963, 1974, 1976). Klare also discusses the methodology of constructing these formulae. For present purposes it is sufficient to know that readability formulae are essentially regression equations for predicting difficulty of text from such predictors as word length, sentence length, and frequency of occurrence in written language as a whole of the words used in the text being measured. In general it would be expected that polysyllabic words will be harder to comprehend than words with fewer syllables. Similarly it would be expected that longer sentences would be harder to understand than shorter sentences. Further it would be expected that rare words would be harder to understand than words in common use.

There is considerable evidence to show that readability scores derived from the formulae to be described have several correlates of interest (Klare, 1963, 1974, 1976; Ley, 1977). These include:

(a) standardised reading tests;
(b) the speed with which a passage can be read;
(c) judgements of difficulty of text;
(d) the probability that an article in a newspaper will be read;
(e) knowledge of content after reading the text.

Thus, the higher the readability the faster text can be read; and the greater will be the probability that it will in fact be read, that it will be judged easy to read, and that readers will be able to answer questions about it.

The formulae most often used in research into the understandability of written health-related information have been the Flesch Formula (Flesch 1948); the Dale–Chall Formula (Dale and Chall, 1948a,b); and the SMOG Grading (McLaughlin, 1969). SMOG stands for Simple Measure of Gobbledygook.

The first of these, the Flesch Formula, reads as follows:

$$\text{Reading Ease} = 206.835 - 0.846W - 1.015S$$

where: W = average number of syllables per hundred words;
S = average number of words in a sentence.

Thus the Flesch formula measures text difficulty by reference to word length and sentence length. To use the formula samples of 100 words of text are taken at random from the document being examined. Reading Ease is calculated for each passage so selected, and the average Reading Ease computed. (In the case of relatively short documents word and sentence lengths can be assessed for the whole text.) The value so obtained is then interpreted by reference to a table, which gives a verbal description of the difficulty level, the US school grade which should have been completed for understanding of the written material, and an estimate of the population likely to understand material at that level of difficulty. This last figure will vary as a function of the percentage of the population who successfully complete the different grade levels, and so will vary with changes in the percentage of students staying on at school and similar factors. For example, the percentage of the US population aged over 25 years who were high school graduates rose from 55 per cent in 1970 to 68 per cent in 1979 (US Department of Commerce, 1980). These sorts of changes make any interpretation for the population as a whole even more hazardous than it would normally be.

Table 8.3 is a rough guide to the interpretation of Reading Ease Scores. The table is derived in part from Flesch (1948) and from data on the percentage of US inhabitants over age 25 who had completed a given number of years of education as revealed by the 1979 census figures (US Department of Commerce, 1980). Because of the relatively rapid changes in educational attainments referred to above, data are provided for (a) all aged over 25 years, and (b) those aged over 65 years. Also followed in constructing the table is Flesch's suggestion that the best estimate of the percentage likely to understand is probably the percentage achieving one grade above the cut-off

Table 8.3: Interpretation of Flesch Reading Ease Scores

Reading Ease Score	Verbal description	Typical text	Completed grade level required to understand	Estimated percentage who would understand	
				aged 25+	aged 65+
90–100	Very easy	Comics	4	97	91
80–90	Easy	Pulp fiction	5	95	88
70–80	Fairly easy	Slick fiction	6	90	77
60–70	Standard	Digests	7–8		
50–60	Fairly hard	Quality	Some high school	77	50
30–50	Difficult	Academic	High school or some college	31	17
0–30	Very hard	Scientific	College	7	3

grade corresponding to a given Reading Ease Score. This suggestion seems very reasonable in the light of findings such as those of Doak and Doak (1980), who administered a standardised reading test (WRAT) to a sample of 100 patients attending a public hospital in Virginia. In this group of patients actual reading ability was on average four to five grades behind the grade completed at school. This reinforces the point that the estimate obtained by use of the Flesch Formula and Table 8.3 is inevitably subject to error, and should therefore be treated only as a rough guide. A further problem arises when attempting to transfer the results from one country to another. However, there is considerable evidence that readability indices have validity in countries other than the USA and in languages other than English (e.g. Ley and Morris, 1984; Ley *et al.*, 1985; Wagenaar, Schreuder and Wijlhuizen, 1987).

Another point, which cannot be emphasised too much, is that whereas low readability almost certainly means that there is something wrong, a score indicating high readability does not mean that all is well. An adequate readability score is a necessary but not sufficient indicator of a good written communication. Unfortunately good readability scores can be obtained by documents written in appalling style, and by documents with poorly chosen content. Nevertheless a poor score does indicate that something is amiss, and that the written material needs simplifying.

The Dale–Chall Formula is based on sentence length and a measure of frequency of use of common words. The formula reads as follows:

Estimated Grade Level $= 0.1579D + 0.0496S + 3.6365$

where D = percentage of words not in Dale's list of 3000 words;

S = average number of words per sentence.

The formula yields an estimate of the grade level needed to understand the text in question. The Dale List of 3000 words can be found in Dale and Chall (1948b). As this formula and the SMOG Index require data on the percentage of the US population who have completed various grades these are shown in Table 8.4. Once more because of the changes in educational attainments over the last decades data are presented separately

Table 8.4: Percentage of US population completing various years of schooling

Years of school completed	Grade	Percentage of over-25s	Percentage of over-65s
Elementary school			
4 or less	4–	3.5	9.2
5	5	1.3	3.4
6–7	6–7	4.9	10.7
8	8	8.6	20.9
High school			
1	9	4.2	5.6
2	10	5.6	6.6
3	11	4.2	3.6
4	12	36.6	23.3
College			
1		5.3	2.8
2		6.8	4.0
3		2.6	1.6
4		9.4	5.2
5 or more		7.0	3.3

for the group aged 25+ and for the group aged 65+.

The third formula to be described is the SMOG Grading. To use this technique it is necessary to select three groups of ten consecutive sentences. One from the beginning, one from the middle, and one from the end of the text to be analysed. The next step is to count the number of words containing three or more syllables (polysyllable count). The square root of this value is then added to 3 to obtain the SMOG Grading. Thus the formula reads as follows:

SMOG Grading = 3 + the square root of the polysyllable count

where:
polysyllable count = number of words of three or more syllables in the 30 sentences;
SMOG Grading = estimated school grade required for understanding the text.

In general it seems that these and other readability measures correlate quite well with one another (Klare, 1974). However, this means simply that the formulae are consistent in ranking text in order of difficulty. Much more important in the present context is the question of whether they yield similar estimates of absolute level of difficulty. Morris, Myers and Thilman (1980) investigated this problem using as text four different versions of a leaflet about valium. Thirteen formulae were applied to these written materials including the Flesch, Dale–Chall and SMOG formulae. The results showed that all formulae ranked the four texts in exactly the same order of difficulty. Unfortunately estimated grade levels required for understanding were not so consistent. Thus the grade estimates in relation to the easiest of the four leaflets ranged from Grade 3 to Grade 8. In the case of the most difficult leaflet, estimates ranged from Grade 5 to College Graduate. Despite this overall variability, however, results given by the Flesch, Dale–Chall and SMOG techniques were very consistent. Eight of the twelve estimates yielded exactly the same grade, and the average difference between estimates was 0.76 of a grade. As there is a great deal of evidence attesting to the external validity of the Flesch and Dale–Chall formulae the findings of Morris *et al.* can be interpreted as supporting the use of these formulae rather than some of their competitors. Nevertheless the differences reported should reinforce the warning, given earlier, that readability formulae should only be used as a rough guide.

THE UNDERSTANDABILITY OF WRITTEN INFORMATION FOR PATIENTS AS ASSESSED BY READABILITY FORMULAE

Investigations of the understandability of health- and welfare-related written materials intended for the lay person have included studies of information for diabetics (Thrush and Lanese, 1962); X-ray leaflets (Ley *et al.*, 1972); dental leaflets for children (Ley, 1973); patient package inserts (Pyrczak and Roth, 1976; Liguori, 1978; Holcomb, 1983); ophthalmic leaflets (French, Mellor and Parry, 1978); health education materials (Cole, 1979); informed consent forms (Grundner, 1980; Morrow, 1980); behaviour therapy self-help manuals (Andrasik and Murphy, 1977; O'Farrell and Keuther, 1983); welfare leaflets (Bendick and Cantu, 1978); written information about cancer (Department of Health, Education and Welfare, 1979); a hundred leaflets and forms about a wide range of medical topics issued by a Virginia hospital (Doak and Doak, 1980); and warning labels (Ley *et al.*, 1985). The results of most of these investigations are summarised in Table 8.5.

Not included in the table are the investigations by Andrasik and Murphy, because their sample of texts probably included some not really intended for a non-professional audience. Morrow's investigation is not in Table 8.5 either, because the data were not reported in suitable form. Morrow examined 60 informed consent leaflets and found them to have a mean Reading Ease Score of 41. Further, 61 per cent of the samples of text used in deriving the Reading Ease Score were at a level of difficulty requiring college education for their understanding. Thus Morrow's findings are consistent with the rest in showing that a great deal of written material produced for patients is likely to be too difficult for them to understand. In an interesting comparison Morrow reported that the mean Reading Ease Score for a sample of medical journals was 34, not much different from the mean of 41 for the informed consent forms. Also excluded are the data of Holcomb, which used the cloze procedure (Taylor, 1953) and those of Ley *et al.* (1985) which studied only two warning labels. (The cloze procedure is a very

Table 8.5: Readability of health and welfare related written materials

Investigations	Number of documents obtaining Flesch Reading Ease Score or equivalent of:					
	80+	70–80	60–70	50–60	30–50	0–30
(a) *Using Flesch Formula*						
Ley *et al.* (1972)	—	—	3	2	—	—
Ley (1973)	—	1	2	1	1	—
French *et al.* (1978)	—	—	9	20	7	—
Liguori (1978)	—	2	—	1	1	—
Cole (1979)	—	2	3	2	2	—
Grundner (1980)	—	—	—	—	1	4
O'Farrell and Keuther (1983)	2	8	44	47	22	1
(b) *Using SMOG Grading*						
Dept. of Health, Education and Welfare (1979)	—	—	2	7	11	1
Doak and Doak (1980)	1	2	21	46	29	1
(c) *Using Dale–Chall Formula*						
Thrush and Lanese (1962)	2	1	6	5	1	1
Pyrczak and Roth (1976)	—	—	—	4	5	1
Bendick and Cantu (1978)	(	11	)	22	(	50	)

useful technique for experimental purposes, but it does not easily lend itself to estimating the proportion of the population who would be expected to understand text.)

Of the leaflets and other documents measured in the investigations summarised in Table 8.5, excluding the welfare materials of Bendick and Cantu, about a quarter would require college education for easy understanding and thus would *not* be understood by approximately 70 per cent of those aged 25 and over, and by 83 per cent of those aged over 65. Further about a quarter of the over-25s and half the over-65s would *not* be able to understand half of these written materials. The findings for the welfare booklets are similar; 60 per cent of these would be estimated to be too difficult for 70 per cent of over-25s and 83 per cent of over-65s. A quarter of the over-25s and half the over-65s would find 87 per cent of these leaflets too difficult. These estimates of percentages likely to understand might well be too generous. Thus in the investigation by Doak and Doak (1980) it was found that 20 per cent of their patient sample had difficulty with Grade 5 material, and a further 60 per cent had reading ability at the 7th to 8th Grade level. As over 75 per cent of the written information issued to these patients required reading ability at the 9th Grade or higher, it would be expected that most of the leaflets and other materials, issued to those patients, would be well beyond the comprehension of most of them.

While it cannot be claimed that the written materials included in the studies reviewed are necessarily a representative sample of such materials in general, it seems likely that considerable numbers of leaflets and other documents for patients are at too high a difficulty level. The moral is obvious. Anyone producing written information for patients should routinely apply a readability formula to it. If readability is low then the material should be re-written.

RECALL OF WRITTEN MATERIAL

The research into patients' recall of medical information, which was reviewed earlier, has included several studies of recall of written information. This has been concerned with patients' recall of informed consent to drug and surgical procedures (Morrow, Gootnick and Schmale, 1978; Bergler *et al.*, 1980;

Cassileth *et al.*, 1980); information about gout (Moll and Wright, 1972; Moll, Wright, Jeffrey, Goode and Humberstone, 1977); mixed medical information (Ley and Spelman, 1967); information about X-ray examination (Ley *et al.*, 1972); and obesity, (Bradshaw et al., 1975). The results of this research are shown in Table 8.6.

Because of the differences in methodology some caution should be exercised in making comparisons between the percentages recalled by those receiving written information and the recall rates reported earlier for recall of orally presented information. Thus, for example, Moll and Wright (1972), Bergler *et al.* (1980), and Cassileth *et al.* (1980) used a multiple choice test of recall. With four alternatives this would lead to a chance score of 25 per cent on average for a patient who in reality could recall nothing. Obviously this chance factor will have had the effect of inflating estimates of percentages recalled in these studies. Fortunately the investigations by Ley and Spelman (1967) and Bradshaw *et al.* (1975) allowed direct comparison of rates of recall for material presented orally or in writing. In these studies no differences emerged in percentage recalled for the two different modes of presentation. It is therefore likely that no reduction in recall will occur if written material is used alone (provided of course, that the patient reads it), and, as reported above, Ellis *et al.* (1979) found that when it is used to supplement oral presentation recall is better.

Table 8.6: Recall of written medical information

Investigation	Time between presentation and recall	Mean percentage recalled
(a) *Informed consent studies*		
Morrow *et al.* (1978)	<5 minutes	74
Bergler *et al.* (1980)	(a) 2 hours	72
	(b) 3 months	62
Cassileth *et al.* (1980)	<1 day	69
(b) *Clinical studies*		
Moll and Wright (1972)	1 week–3 years	60
Moll *et al.* (1977)	'routine follow-up period'	66
(c) *Analogue studies*		
Ley and Spelman (1967)	1 hour	44
Ley *et al.* (1972)	(a) 20 minutes	76
	(b) 20 minutes	69
Bradshaw *et al.* (1975)	(a) <1 minute	28
	(b) <1 minute	34

In addition the written material can in theory be used for later reference. In practice this seems to happen; for example, Kanouse *et al.* (1981) found that of those receiving leaflets about erythromycin, nitrazepam, and oestrogens, the respective percentages reporting that they kept the leaflets for future reference were 54, 57 and 45 per cent. Further, 32, 22 and 29 per cent, respectively, claimed to have actually read their leaflet more than once, as did 72 per cent of the patients studied by Moll and Wright (1972).

The conclusion is therefore that patients do indeed forget much of the written material presented to them, but that by its nature written information has the advantage of being available for refreshing one's memory, and it seems that patients take advantage of this.

SUMMARY

We have seen that written information can often be of use in clinical settings, either on its own or as an adjunct to orally presented information. Problems involved in the use of written materials include the following:

(a) they are not always noticed;
(b) they are not always read;
(c) they are not always understood; and
(d) they are not always remembered.

It is therefore likely that written information could be improved in various ways. The next chapter will examine the success of attempts to achieve these improvements.

9

The Improvement of Written Information

INTRODUCTION

This chapter will describe research into ways of increasing the probability that the written material will be noticed, read, understood, believed and remembered.

There is virtually no evidence available concerning factors determining whether health-related written information will be noticed, or read. Presumably a lot will depend on whether the leaflet is actually given by the clinician to the patient or whether it is left on display in a container labelled: 'Please take one of these leaflets'. In the first case it would be very hard for the patient not to notice the leaflet, in the second it would be much easier. Certainly it cannot be taken for granted that significant information will be noticed. Ley *et al.* (1985) found that approximately 50 per cent of keyboard and secretarial staff, who regularly used erasing fluid, were unaware that there was a warning label on the fluid's container. It is therefore necessary to make sure that the audience's attention is called to the written information provided.

The next problem is to see that the material is read. As we have seen, while the majority of patients claim to have read the information given to them, on average about 30 per cent claim not to have done so. There appears to be little research in health-related contexts on the effectiveness of attempts to make material more attractive by the use of colour cartoons, and illustrations in increasing the percentage of recipients of written information who claim to have read it. However, some research has been conducted into the effects of these and similar variables on recall and knowledge of content of leaflets. In non-clinical contexts increasing readability has been shown to increase the probability that a piece of writing will be read (Klare, 1963, 1976).

However, the usual aim of increasing readability is to increase the understandability of the material. Increases in readability can most easily be achieved by the use of shorter words and shorter sentences. It should be noted that it is necessary to make *both* of these changes for there to be a likely increase in comprehension (Klare, 1976). In addition Klare found that the change in readability should be large to produce results. Thus the mean change in grade level in studies reporting significant effects was 6.5 grades, whereas in those reporting no effect or mixed results it was 4.25 grades.

Kanouse and Hayes-Roth (1980) have suggested other ways in which the comprehensibility of text can be increased. These suggestions were based on a review of experimental psychological laboratory studies of understandability of text. The suggestions include:

(a) using the active rather than the passive voice;
(b) filling subject, verb, and object positions with important content words, not fillers, i.e. avoid 'there are', 'it is thought', etc.;
(c) using concrete rather than abstract words and sentences;
(d) using consistent terminology to refer to common referents;
(e) stating presuppositions explicitly before referring to them implicitly;
(f) putting new information at the end of a sentence and old information at the beginning;
(g) not deleting pronouns or clause markers;
(h) using numbering or bulleting to present facts in a paragraph;
(i) using clear markers of time and cause and effect;
(j) using relatively short sentences.

Kanouse and Hayes-Roth were of course quite aware that the transfer of findings from the laboratory to the field is often a disappointing exercise, and as we shall see they put some of these principles to the test in the Rand Corporation investigation (Kanouse *et al.*, 1981a,b). Similar recommendations are made in the review edited by Felker (1980).

Increasing the memorability of text should in theory be achievable by increasing comprehensibility, so the factors just discussed should also affect memory. In addition the variables earlier shown to improve memory for orally presented information would also be expected to increase recall of written information, e.g. explicit categorisation, repetition, and use of specific advice statements.

It would also be expected that the physical packaging of written information might make a difference to the probability of its being noticed, read, understood and remembered. Several reviews are available describing this research in some detail (Tinker, 1963; 1966; Poulton, 1969; Wright, 1977; 1978; 1983; MacDonald-Ross, 1978; Hartley, 1980; 1982; Felker, 1980). Some of these have been summarised by Poulton, Warren and Bond (1970) whose list includes the following:

(a) unjustified lines are easier to read;
(b) type should be at least 10 point;
(c) leading is probably unnecessary;
(d) indenting the first line of a paragraph increases speed of reading;
(e) titles all in capitals are harder to pick out;
(f) printing in capitals reduces speed of comprehension;
(g) printing in italics reduces speed of reading;
(h) headings should be made to stand out by the use of a different type face or by the use of space;
(i) arabic numerals are read more quickly than roman numerals.

This list gives the flavour of many of the suggestions for improving leaflet design which can be derived from experimental studies. Advice about graphics is harder to summarise. It is known that the use of illustrations is not always an aid to understanding (e.g. Dwyer, 1971, 1972; Snowman and Cunningham, 1975; Willows, 1978). The conditions under which graphical aids will be effective are not known with any certainty.

127

EFFECTIVENESS OF ATTEMPTS TO IMPROVE WRITTEN INFORMATION BY INCREASING READABILITY

The most frequently reported method of attempting to improve written information for patients has been to try to increase its understandability and then assess the effects of this manipulation on patients' recall and compliance. The most obvious way to investigate this problem is by comparisons of the effectiveness of materials differing in readability. Klare (1976) reviewed 36 experimental studies of the effects of manipulating the readability of non-health-related materials, and found that in 19 studies increased readability improved comprehension, in 6 studies it had mixed results, and in 11 studies it had no effect. In further analyses of these investigations Klare isolated a number of variables associated with whether or not an increase in readability led to an increase in comprehension; including reader competence, reader motivation and content of the material. An increase in readability is less likely to increase comprehension:

(a) the higher the reading ability of the reader;
(b) the higher the motivation of the reader;
(c) the higher the interest of the content of the material to the reader; and,
(d) the amount the reader already knows about the topic.

On the face of it some of these variables might be likely to reduce the benefits of increasing the readability of written information for patients. On the basis of the survey and interview studies reviewed earlier, it would obviously be expected that patients would be highly motivated to acquire, and be interested in, information about their condition and its treatment. Add to this the fact that the material presented will often be a very short booklet or leaflet, and it will be seen that it is not self evident that increasing readability will increase comprehension, memory or compliance in this highly motivated and interested audience. Further, patients with chronic of often repeated illnesses might over time acquire a considerable amount of information about their illnesses, and so there would be little chance of the readability of written materials affecting their knowledge.

Klare also considered another possible danger in increasing readability. This is that by making material too easy it will become unsuitable or unacceptable to the more intelligent reader. Klare concluded that in general the evidence does not support this possibility. Finally, it is worth recalling that Klare found that increases in readability of relatively small magnitude were less likely to lead to increased comprehension than larger changes in readability. As we shall see some of the changes in experiments in the clinical area have been quite small.

The effects of changing the readability of health-related leaflets have been reported by Ley *et al.* (1972, 1975a, 1979, 1985); Bradshaw *et al.* (1975); Eaton and Holloway (1980); Ley (1982a, 1987a). Topics covered by these leaflets consisted of information about: (a) X-ray investigations; (b) weight reducing diets; (c) anti-depressant and tranquillising medication; (d) the menopause; (e) warfarin medication; (f) glaucoma; (g) the dangers of inhaling volatile substances; and (h) antibiotic medication.

Ley *et al.* (1972) randomly assigned 90 subjects to the task of recalling the content of one of three versions of two leaflets. One leaflet described the procedures involved in a barium meal X-ray examination and instructed the patient about how to prepare for it. The second leaflet performed the same tasks with respect to a cholecystogram. In each case the control leaflet was the one normally used in the hospital where the research was conducted. The modifications consisted of (a) increasing readability by shortening words and sentences, and (b) using the same modified text but inserting headings. The insertion of headings made no difference to recall of either leaflet. Increasing readability had no effect on knowledge of contents of the barium meal leaflet, but had the predicted effect on knowledge of the cholecystogram leaflet.

The effect of a change in readability on recall of instructions about a weight-reduction programme were investigated by Bradshaw *et al.* (1975). In the first experiment 40 subjects were randomly assigned to learning either easy or hard material. (Easy material had a Flesch Reading Ease Score of 90 or more, and hard material a score of 25 or less.) In the second experiment, 32 subjects received a mixture of hard and easy statements to recall. In the first experiment there were no significant differences in recall between those receiving the hard and easy statements, whereas in the second experiment the easy statements were better recalled. Note, however, that in these experiments subjects read written statements aloud, which is somewhat different from the usual way in which a patient would deal with such material.

Ley *et al.* (1975a) investigated the effect of changes in the readability of a medication leaflet on the accuracy with which depressed and anxious patients took their medicine. Interviews with patients had revealed that many were not aware that tranquillisers and anti-depressants took some time to exert their effects, and that there was considerable confusion about what to do if by chance a dose was forgotten. Two leaflets, one for the anti-depressant and one for the tranquillising medications, which gave information about these problems, were prepared by an experienced clinician. As might be expected from the evidence reviewed above these proved gratifyingly difficult producing Reading Ease Scores of 18 and 23 respectively. Two easier versions of these leaflets were then prepared, one with a score between 55 and 70, and one with a score between 90 and 100. The subjects of this research were 80 consecutive depressed and 80 consecutive anxious patients who met the criterion of having only one medicine prescribed for them. Within each group patients were randomly assigned to receiving either (a) no leaflet, (b) the hard leaflet, (c) the moderately hard leaflet, or (d) the easy leaflet. An accuracy of medicine-taking score, derived by dividing the difference between the number of tablets taken and the number which should have been taken, by the number which should have been taken showed significant decreases in medication errors with increases in the readability of the written information to which the patients were exposed. Thus the easy leaflet produced fewer errors than the moderately hard leaflet, which in turn produced fewer errors than the hard leaflet, which in fact was no better than not receiving a leaflet at all. The importance of this study lies particularly in its demonstration that the effectiveness of providing written information is likely to depend on the readability of that information.

A booklet giving information about the menopause was the material used in the investigation by Ley *et al.* (1979). A total of 72 women general practice patients, expected shortly to enter the menopause, were randomly assigned to receiving the booklet normally used in that practice or a modified version with higher readability. Women receiving the version with the higher readability had significantly more knowledge of the content when tested at a follow-up visit.

Eaton and Holloway (1980) assigned 108 outpatients at a

Minnesota Veterans Administration hospital, who were not being treated with warfarin sodium, to receiving a pamphlet about this drug, written at either 5th grade or 10th grade level. Patients receiving the 5th grade level material showed significantly better knowledge of content than those who received the 10th grade material. Eaton and Holloway also investigated the question of whether increased readability would be of more benefit to those with poorer reading skills. To their surprise they found no evidence that this was so. These investigators used the Raygor Readability Estimate to assess readability.

Ley (1982a) studied undergraduate subjects' recall of written information about glaucoma. The students were randomly assigned to receiving either a hard or an easy version of a leaflet describing the symptomatology, aetiology, treatment and prognosis of glaucoma. Students assigned to the easier version retained significantly more of the content than those receiving the hard version. This study is of interest in showing that differences in readability of medical information can exert an effect even on a young audience of higher intelligence.

The problem of the effect of differences in the readability of warning labels about the dangers of deliberately inhaling volatile substances was investigated in three experiments, by Ley et al. (1985). In all experiments subjects were randomly assigned to reading either a hard or an easy version of the warning. The hard version was judged as being at 9th grade level by the Flesch Formula, and the easy one at 5th grade level. In the first experiment subjects consisted of school students in Grades 5 to 11. In the second experiment the subjects attending meetings of Parent–Teacher Associations. In the third experiment the subjects were secretaries and office workers. Increased readability led to significantly greater knowledge of contents in the school and secretarial groups, but not in the parent group. Further, this effect was most pronounced amongst students in the 5th and 6th Grades. In addition, it was found that those reading the easier label were more likely to say that they understood and, in the case of the younger students, that they believed the warning.

Finally, Ley (1987a) studied the effect of differences in readability on the time taken to read a leaflet about erythromycin, and on recall of its contents. Subjects were all over age 65, and it was found that the easiest version was (a) read faster, and (b) better recalled than the two harder versions.

The results of these studies are summarised in Table 9.1 in which the percentage improvement measure is derived by taking the difference between the experimental condition and the control condition, and expressing the value so found as a percentage of the control value. The numbers in the column headed 'Difference in grade' are the difference in grades between the grade level of the experimental and control materials. All the studies reported in Table 9.1, except for that of Eaton and Holloway, used the Flesch Formula to assess the readability of the materials involved, so where Flesch assigned a range of grade levels to the Reading Ease Score interval in which the score in question falls, some discretion has been exercised in assigning a grade level to it. Scores at the top of the

Table 9.1: Effects of increasing the readability of medical information

Investigation	Topic		Percentage improvement	Difference in grade level	p
Studies of memory — comprehension					
Ley *et al.* (1972)	(a) barium meal X-ray		−6	3	n.s.
	(b) cholecystogram		+34	4	<0.01
Bradshaw *et al.* (1975)	Weight-reducing diet instructions	(a)	+29	8	n.s.
		(b)	+72	8	<0.05
Ley *et al.* (1979)	Menopause information		+22	2	<0.05
Eaton and Holloway (1980)	Warfarin medication		—	5	<0.001
Ley (1982a)	Glaucoma information		+34	2	<0.001
Ley *et al.* (1985)	Warning about danger of inhaling volatile substances				
	(a) Grades 5 and 6		+126	4	<0.001
	(b) Grades 9–11		+45	4	<0.001
	(c) Parents		+14	4	n.s.
	(d) Secretaries		+48	4	<0.01
Ley (1987a)	Antibiotic information				
	(1) recall	(a)	+116	3	<0.01
		(b)	+128	6	<0.01
	(2) reading speed	(a)	+29	3	<0.01
		(b)	+24	6	<0.01
Studies of compliance					
Ley *et al.* (1975a)	(a) Tranquillising medication	(a)	+47	8	<0.05
		(b)	+61	12	<0.05
	(b) Anti-depressant medication	(a)	+44	6	<0.05
		(b)	+82	12	<0.05

range have been assigned the lowest grade corresponding to that range, scores in the middle of the range the median grade corresponding to that range, and so on. Lastly, Eaton and Holloway did not report their results in a form which permits the entry of a value in the 'Percentage improvement' column. It can be seen that, despite the probably high motivation of the subjects, and the probably high level of interest of the materials for them, an increase in readability often has desirable results.

EFFECTIVENESS OF OTHER METHODS OF IMPROVING WRITTEN INFORMATION

In addition to increasing readability investigators have attempted to increase the effectiveness of written information by increasing its comprehensibility and memorability in other ways. These have included (a) the use of specific rather than general statements (Bradshaw *et al.*, 1975; Berry *et al.*, 1981; Kanouse *et al.*, 1981a,b; Winkler *et al.*, 1981); (b) mixture of increased readability, explicit categorisation and repetition (Ley, 1978; Ley *et al.*, 1979); (c) mixture of increased readability, use of the active voice, avoidance of negatives and technical terms (Berry *et al.*, 1981; Kanouse *et al.*, 1981; Winkler *et al.*, 1981); (d) use of adjunct questions (Ley and Morris, 1984); (e) use of primacy effects (Ley and Morris, 1984).

The effect of making instructions more specific was investigated by Bradshaw *et al.* (1975), who found that specific advice statements about a weight-reducing diet were significantly better recalled than more generally phrased statements, thus echoing their finding about the recall of orally presented advice statements. However, Berry *et al.* (1981), Kanouse *et al.* (1981) and Winkler *et al.* (1981) did not find that specificity affected either knowledge or compliance. Interpretation of these different findings is complicated by the fact that whereas the subjects of Bradshaw *et al.* received between 5 and 20 statements to recall after only one reading, those of the other investigators received much more material than this, but could read it more than once if they wished, with 22–32 per cent claiming to have done this.

Studies of the effectiveness of mixtures of increased readability, explicit categorisation, and repetition have been reported by Ley (1978), and Ley *et al.* (1979). In the first of these the effects of using this mixture of techniques to increase the effectiveness of a booklet advising obese females about procedures to lose weight were investigated. Three experiments were reported, in each of which a standard booklet was compared with a modified booklet. In the first experiment a highly statistically and clinically significant result was obtained. At 8 week follow-up women receiving the modified booklet had lost, on average, 5.58 kg as compared with the 3.49 kg lost by those receiving the standard booklet. Unfortunately two repetitions of this experiment failed to confirm this impressive result. In a study of a different topic area, Ley et al. (1979) compared general practice patients' knowledge levels after they had read either a standard booklet about contraception or a modified one. No differences in knowledge were found between the groups receiving the different booklets.

The mixture of techniques used in the Rand Corporation study to increase the comprehensibility of the leaflets involved included the use of the active voice, shorter sentences, fewer technical words, and fewer negatives. These modifications did not have any effects on knowledge or compliance with the flurazepam, the oestrogen, or the erythromycin leaflets (Berry et al., 1981; Kanouse et al., 1981a,b; Winkler et al., 1981).

An investigation of the usefulness of using primacy effects to control differential recall of the content of different sections of a leaflet giving information about glaucoma was conducted by Ley (1982a). Although a primacy effect was found, in that the first few statements presented were better recalled, this effect was not strong enough to affect overall recall of sections consisting of several statements.

Finally, Ley (1982a) attempted to increase the knowledge gained from reading a leaflet about childhood illness by the use of adjunct questions. (Adjunct questions are questions about content presented either at the beginning or end of the material.) The attempt was unsuccessful.

The results of these investigations are shown in Table 9.2. Note that in the summary of the data presented by Berry et al. no single summary statistic is presented for compliance, so data on two measures are provided.

Perhaps the most remarkable feature of this table is the very large number of negative results. At first glance the most surprising finding is that mixtures consisting of increased readability plus other supposedly comprehension- and memory-

Table 9.2: Effects on knowledge and compliance of attempts to increase the comprehensibility of written information

Investigation	Material	Modification	Percentage change	p
(a) Knowledge				
Bradshaw *et al.* (1975)	Weight-reduction instructions	Use of specific statements	(a)+339 (b)+187	<0.001 <0.001
Berry *et al.* (1981)	Flurazepam leaflet	(a) Use of specific statements	−4	n.s.
		(b) Mixture	+1	n.s.
Kanouse *et al.* (1981)	Oestrogen leaflet	(a) Use of specific statements	−2	n.s.
		(b) Mixture	−1	n.s.
Winkler *et al* (1981)	Erythromycin leaflet	(a) Use of specific statements	+1	n.s.
		(b) Mixture	+4	n.s.
Ley *et al.* (1979)	Contraception booklet	Mixture	−6	n.s.
Ley (1982c)	Glaucoma leaflet	Primacy	0	n.s.
Ley (1982d)	Pediatric	Adjunct questions	−20	n.s.
(b) Compliance				
Ley (1978)	Weight-reducing booklet	Mixture	(a) +60 (b) −10 (c) −4	<0.01 n.s. n.s.
Berry *et al.* (1981)	Flurazepam leaflet	(a) Use of specific statements needed tablet not taken	+7	n.s.
		unnecessary tablet taken	−28	n.s.
		(b) Mixture needed tablet not taken	+17	n.s.
		unnecessary tablet taken	+26	n.s.
Kanouse *et al.* (1981)	Oestrogen leaflet	(a) Use of specific statements	+6	n.s.
		(b) Mixture	−2	n.s.
Winkler *et al.* (1981)	Erythromycin leaflet	(a) Use of specific statements	−2	n.s.
		(b) Mixture	−5	n.s.

enhancing techniques should have so little effect on knowledge, when increased readability on its own seems to have a positive effect. It is possible that part of the reason for this failure is that the hard and easy versions of leaflets for the three drugs studied by Berry *et al.*; Kanouse *et al.* and Winkler *et al.* only differed by two grade levels as assessed by the SMOG Grading technique. However the Flesch Reading Ease Scores given by Ley *et al.* correspond to a difference of five grade levels. Another possibility is that the opportunity to re-read the leaflets and discuss them with others over-rode the effect of any readability differences. But whatever the reasons, this is a resoundingly negative set of results.

In the Rand Corporation investigation, patients receiving written information at least had greater knowledge than those who received no leaflet. However, Dolinsky, Gross, Deutsch, Demestihas and Dolinsky (1983) found no differences between patients receiving modified leaflets and patients receiving no leaflet. Modifications were similar to those used to increase understandability in the Rand study. This finding lends support to the findings discussed above.

ATTEMPTS TO IMPROVE THE PHYSICAL PACKAGING OF INFORMATION

Investigations of the effect of physical features of written information have been concerned with (a) the use of illustrations; (b) comparisons of outline and narrative formats; and, (c) highlighting of parts of the content of the leaflet.

There are a number of possible dangers in the use of illustrations. Firstly, they might act as distractors, and thus divert attention from the text. Secondly, people often spontaneously develop images which help them comprehend and remember text. Illustrations provided in the text might in some cases be in conflict with these spontaneously produced images and thus reduce their effectiveness. Thirdly, it is possible, in the case of medical information, that some illustrations might be anxiety-provoking or aversive to some of those reading the leaflet containing them. Thus it is not self-evident that illustrations will improve understanding or recall. Indeed in the non-clinical field there is a great deal of evidence to show that the use of illustration has mixed results (Ley and Morris, 1984).

On the other hand it is hard to imagine that some procedures are better described in words than in pictures, e.g. the correct insertion of eye-drops. This is especially true when technical terminology is involved. An excellent example of the superiority of diagram over words can be found in Wright (1977), who presents a clear diagram, which is the graphical equivalent of: 'See that the sliding dog associated with the reverse drive bevel is rotating freely before tightening the long differential casing'.

The use of illustration in attempts to improve the effectiveness of written information has had two main purposes. These are: (a) to increase understanding directly by the use of appropriate diagrams, and (b) to achieve this effect indirectly by making the material more attractive and thus more likely to be read.

A good example of the use of illustration directly to increase understanding can be found in the work of Dwyer (1972). Dwyer experimented with different illustrations of the heart, ranging from full colour photographs to simple line drawings, to assess their effectiveness as aids to understanding heart structure and function. The results showed that simple line drawings were the most effective.

Lovius, Lovius and Ley (1973) also attempted to increase directly the amount of knowledge acquired from an oral hygiene pamphlet by children aged 12 or slightly older. Subjects were tested for knowledge of correct oral hygiene practices before and after reading the leaflet, and also at a three month follow-up. Children were randomly assigned to receiving either text only or the same text plus relevant illustrations. Although the text was effective in improving knowledge, 66 per cent showing increased knowledge at immediate test and 63 per cent three months later, the use of illustrations had no effect on knowledge acquisition.

These last two studies investigated the use of illustration as a supplement to text. However, Hardie, Gagnon and Eckel (1979) assessed the possibility that symbolic diagrams could be used in place of written directions for use of prescribed medication. A major aim of this study was to see if diagrammatic pictorial material would be easier for poorer readers. The directions for use were, in their verbal form, the ten most frequently occurring in the hospital where the investigators worked. For each of the verbal directions a non-verbal pictorial equivalent was devised thus yielding in all 20 directions for use. The subjects of this investigation were 309 patients, who chose to have the prescription filled at the hospital pharmacy. Those who agreed to cooperate in the research, about 90 per cent of those approached, were presented with 20 labels each containing a direction for use. Except for patients at the lowest levels of reading ability, where there was no difference between the two types of direction, the written instructions were better understood. Overall the average patient understood 88 per cent of the written directions and 65 per cent of the graphic directions. At the lowest levels of reading ability, Grade 4 ability or less, 55 per cent of each were understood.

Moll and Wright (1972) and Moll *et al.* (1977) have studied the use of illustrations as indirect aids to increasing knowledge gain from booklets about gout. In fact the illustrations used were cartoons. In the first study patients read a booklet in which some pieces of information were accompanied by cartoons and others not. Nine cartoons were used in all. Recall of the illustrated topics was significantly poorer than recall of unillustrated topics. Simple interpretation of this finding is hampered by the fact that the items accompanied by the cartoons were not varied experimentally, so the findings might simply be a reflection of some pieces of information being harder to learn. The other major alternative hypothesis that the illustrations acted as distractors presumably leads to the prediction that if more cartoons were used knowledge would be even poorer.

The study by Moll *et al.* (1977) provides some help with this problem. In this investigation the illustrated version of the booklet contained 89 cartoons. In addition in this study there was a control group who received an unillustrated version. There were no differences in knowledge between those receiving the two versions, and neither group obtained a significantly greater score on the knowledge test than the group in the investigation of Moll and Wright (1972).

It will also be recalled that Avorn and Sumerai (1983) also found that the use of illustration and colour did not increase the effectiveness of written information in altering the frequency with which physicians prescribed inappropriate or sub-optimal drugs. At best then a verdict of 'not proven' must be brought in concerning the usefulness of adding illustration to written materials for patients.

A number of investigators have inquired into the effects of presenting written materials in note or outline form as opposed to continuous narrative. The largest study of this problem was part of the Rand Corporation investigation. In the case of the oestrogen leaflet (Kanouse *et al.*, 1981), and in the case of the erythromycin leaflet (Winkler *et al.*, 1981), patients were more likely to report having read the outline leaflet. This was not accompanied by higher levels of knowledge in the groups receiving the outline format. However, those receiving the outline were less likely to express willingness to take the drug again, and, in the case of erythromycin, were more likely to report side-effects and health problems. In a different study, Morris and Kanouse (1981) found that recall of information about the side-effects of flurazepam was not affected by whether the information, about these, was in outline or narrative form, in the body of the leaflet.

Berry *et al.* (1981), Kanouse *et al.* (1981) and Winkler *et al.* (1981) also reported that highlighting the risks associated with the drug, by typographical and other cues, did not lead to greater knowledge of those risks. Indeed the only striking effect of highlighting the risks was that oestrogen users who received the leaflets with risks highlighted became more convinced of the drug's effectiveness than other groups (Kanouse *et al.*, 1981).

Morris *et al.* (1977) also found that highlighting risks had disappointingly small effects. These investigators reported that women who were users of oral contraceptives had little idea of what was in a legally required boxed off set of nine warnings to users of these drugs. Fifty-four per cent knew that the danger of blood clots was mentioned in the box, but 87 per cent wrongly thought that the box contained directions for use.

Finally Ley (1987a) investigated elderly people's recall of the content of an antibiotic leaflet. On the basis of some of the research reviewed earlier it was expected that text, all in capitals, would be harder to read and thus lead to poorer recall, and that text in smaller type would be harder than text in larger type. Neither of these expectations was fulfilled. The subjects read and recalled the capitalised and small type texts just as well as the supposedly easier text. However, subjects *ratings* of how hard the text was to read and understand were affected by these changes in format. Material in capitals was rated easier to read, and material in larger type was rated as easier to understand. It will be recalled that in this experiment, as reported above, material rated easy by the Flesch Formula was read faster and recalled better than material with a lower Reading Ease score. Interestingly, variations in Reading Ease had no effect on subjects' ratings.

SUMMARY

There has been little success in attempts to improve the effectiveness of written information for patients. The exception to this gloomy generalisation seems to be that increasing the readability of written materials by shortening words and sentences is effective. At least in the majority of cases material, modified in this way, has proved more effective than control material. Even so, the failure of this technique to work as part of packages of modifications raises some doubts as to the generality of this effect.

However, it is important to remember that, even if there are currently few, if any, certain ways of improving written material, it remains an effective supplement to orally presented information, and is sometimes an effective substitute for it. Even the Rand Corporation Study, which has been the source of so many of the negative results reviewed above, found that patients receiving a leaflet had more knowledge at later test than those who received no leaflet.

10

Selecting the Content of
Communications

INTRODUCTION

This chapter will be concerned with the ways in which the
content of communications to patients can be selected. How do
we decide what topics to cover in an oral or written health-
related message? Possible bases for this decision include:

(a) patients' opinions;
(b) professionals' opinions;
(c) behaviourally defined objectives;
(d) what is needed for rational decision making by patients;
(e) judgemental criteria;
(f) empirical criteria.

These possible options will now be examined in more detail.
Following this a slightly different sort of content question will be
considered. This is the problem of finding potentially motivating
content for the message.

PATIENTS' AND PROFESSIONALS' OPINIONS

When discussing the problem of patients' dissatisfaction with
communications it was pointed out that the majority of patients
appear to want to know as much as possible about their illness
and its treatment. With regard to treatment patients and professionals agree that there are many aspects of their treatment
about which patients should be informed. Nevertheless patients
and health professionals sometimes disagree on the desirability

of information about risks, dangers and other uses being provided to patients. Illustrative data from surveys by Joubert and Lasagna (1975) and Fleckenstein (1977) involving samples of patients, physicians and pharmacists are summarised in Table 10.1.

There is also evidence that at times physicians and the lay population have differed in their opinions about whether patients should be provided with more emotionally charged information. The prime example of this is the question of whether people with cancer or with fatal diseases should be told or not. For many years survey data have shown that the vast majority of the population believe that they should be told if they have cancer or fatal disease (Feiffel, 1963; Ley and Spelman, 1967; Kalish and Reynolds, 1976; Levy, 1983). Until quite recently the majority of physicians thought otherwise. In USA studies, it was reported by Fitts and Ravdin (1953) that 61 per cent of physicians seldom or never told their patients if they had cancer; by Rennick (1960) that 22 per cent never told their

Table 10.1: Opinions of patients, physicians and pharmacists about the desirability of patients being provided with different types of information about their medicines

	Percentage of group thinking that patients should be told		
	Patients (Joubert and Lasagna, 1975)	Physicians (Fleckenstein, 1977)	Pharmacists (Fleckenstein, 1977)
Name of drug	97	92	93
Common risks of normal use	89	85	71
Drugs to avoid when taking this drug	—	81	85
Conditions under which the drug should not be used	—	81	84
Overdose information	86	76	84
Expected benefits	—	69	75
Normal dose range	—	67	61
Risks of using too little	80	52	74
Risks of not using at all	79	46	76
How drug works	—	46	46
All possible benefits of normal use	—	40	30
All possible risks of normal use	77	25	39
Other important uses	75	20	12

142

patients and that only 16 per cent always told them; by Oken (1961) that 90 per cent did not generally inform their patients; and by Friedman (1970) that 25 per cent always told and 9 per cent never told. However, by 1979 it looked as though, at least in the USA, medical attitudes had changed. Novack, Plummer, Smith, Ochtill, Morrow, and Bennett (1979) found that 98 per cent of their sample stated that their usual policy was to tell patients.

It is likely that the reluctance of physicians, pharmacists and other health professionals to provide patients with certain kinds of information is based on the belief that the provision of such information would have adverse effects. In particular the information might cause undue anxiety or distress to patients, or it might decrease compliance with necessary treatment and procedures, or, in the case of medication, lead to more complaint of side-effects. In other words the motivation is one of benevolent paternalism. However, it is probable that patients are much more robust than health care professionals imagine.

EFFECTS OF GIVING INFORMATION WHICH MIGHT CAUSE ADVERSE EFFECTS

A number of investigations have inquired into the effects of providing patients with information of the kind which could, in theory, cause adverse reactions. These have included telling patients that they have cancer; giving patients full access to their case records — and even making them co-authors of these; and telling patients the detailed risks of investigative procedures. Several of these studies are summarised in Table 10.2.

Other studies have investigated the effects of giving patients fuller information about their medication (Myers and Calvert, 1973, 1976, 1978; Newcomer and Anderson, 1974; Eklund and Wessling, 1976; Paulson, Bauch, Paulson and Zilz, 1976; Suveges, 1977; Weibert, 1977; Morris and Kanouse, 1982). All but one of these studies reported no ill effects of giving patients more information. The exception was the study by Newcomer and Anderson which found that the provision of written information about side-effects led more patients to report them. Of particular interest is the study by Morris and Kanouse (1982) who found that the provision of information did not increase the frequency of experiencing side-effects, but did increase the

Table 10.2: Patients' reactions to being given information potentially capable of producing adverse effects

Investigation	Topic	Effect
Kelly and Friesen (1950)	Diagnosis of cancer	89% thought people should be told
Aitken-Swan and Easson (1959)	Diagnosis of cancer	66% thought people should be told
Gilbertsen and Wangensteen (1962)	Diagnosis of cancer	87–93% thought people should be told
Gerle et al. (1960)	Diagnosis of inoperable cancer	Better adjustment than in a group who were not told
Alfidi (1970)	Fully informing patients of the risks of angiographic examination	3% refused examination, 93% thought that patients should be given full information
Greenwood (1973)	Informing mothers of innocent heart murmurs in their children	14% showed anxiety and 5% thought the condition dangerous even after reassurance
Golodetz et al. (1976)	Giving patients access to their case records	4% would have preferred no access
Stevens et al. (1977)	Giving patients access to their case records	No more anxiety or depression than in patients not given access
Fischbach et al. (1980)	Making patient 'co-author of case record	No adverse effects on patients, but took more physician time

probability that they would be attributed to the taking of the drug. Finally a study by Keown, cited by Slovic, Fischoff and Lichtenstein (1980) found that people wanted to know about the serious side effects of drugs such as blood clots and liver damage, even if their frequency of occurrences was as low as once in every 10 000 000 users.

It would seem fair to conclude from this brief review that the predicted or potential adverse reactions to giving patients full information do not often occur. In general people want to know even when the news is bad. In view of this it would seem sensible to provide patients with the information which they say that they would like.

BEHAVIOURALLY DEFINED OBJECTIVES

This approach asks what are the exact medication-related behaviours that the patient needs to exhibit for the proper use of the medication. When this list of behaviours has been constructed it can be used as a basis for deciding what information will be required for the patient to be able to show those behaviours. An excellent example of this approach is provided by Hermann, Herxheimer and Lionel (1978) who list the main categories of behaviour required as:

(a) to know how to take the drug:
    (1) to take a specific dose;
    (2) to take a dose in a specific manner;
    (3) to take a dose at a specific time;
(b) to know how to store the drug:
    (1) to store it properly;
    (2) to recognise the time at which the medicine becomes subpotent;
(c) to know how the drug is expected to help:
    (1) to recall the basic facts about the complaint;
    (2) to recognise the desired effect and act upon its absence;
(d) to recognise problems caused by the drug:
    (1) to recognise unwanted effects if they do occur;
    (2) to recall that certain effects can only be detected by clinical examination or tests;
    (3) to recall circumstances indicating a need for change of treatment and act if they occur;
    (4) to verify components of the medicine;
    (5) to act if overdosage occurs.

The reader can see how this classification immediately provides pointers as to what information needs to be provided. Thus in order to take the drug properly the patient will need to know the amount to be taken, the manner in which the drug is to be taken, e.g. with meals, and the times when the drug should be taken. In their paper Hermann *et al.* provide details of the categories of information which might be needed as well as a 'model' leaflet giving information concerning tetracyclines. The leaflet proposed can, however, be criticised on the grounds that it might well be too difficult for many patients, but as we have seen it is possible to do something about difficulty levels (see Chapter 9).

INFORMATION NEEDED FOR RATIONAL DECISION MAKING BY PATIENTS

Ley (1982b) raised the possibility that it might be worth considering the patient's decision about whether or not to take a medicine, or undergo a particular treatment, in the form of a 'pay-off' matrix. This is a technical term taken from scientific studies of decision-making and refers to a table in which the rows are the possible courses of action available to the person who has to make the decision, 'choices', the columns are the 'events' which could occur following the decision, and the cells in the body of the matrix are the 'outcomes', i.e. combinations of choices and events.

A concrete (somewhat over-simplified) example will probably help. Suppose we wished to lose weight and, further, that we wished to lose a minimum of 9 kg, and would regard losing anything less than this as a waste of time and effort. Assume further that our own unaided efforts have been unsuccessful, and that we are therefore seeking professional help. We are offered a choice between three treatments, (a) anorectic drugs, (b) a behaviour modification package, and (c) a behavioural package combined with a very low calorie diet. The events are that either we lose the 9 kg or we do not. This gives us the matrix shown in Figure 10.1.

It can be seen that there are six cells in the pay-off matrix, each one indicating a combination of a treatment choice and an event. In order to make a 'rational' decision it is necessary to assign weightings to these various outcomes. Let us decide to assign values between −100 and +100. These values are called 'utilities'. Positive values are assigned to desirable combinations and negative values to undesirable ones. The best combination would probably be successfully to lose the weight as a result of taking medication, as this would have involved little time, little cost, and little inconvenience. So let us assign a value of +100 to this outcome. If weight was not lost as a result of medication then this would obviously be undesirable but again little time, little effort and little cost would have been involved. So let us assign a value of −50 to this combination. The behaviour

Figure 10.1: Outline hypothetical pay-off matrix showing the possible choices, events and outcomes for the obesity example

Treatment choices   Events

	Weight lost	Weight not lost
Medication	outcome 1	outcome 2
Behaviour modification	outcome 3	outcome 4
Behaviour modification plus very low calorie diet	outcome 5	outcome 6

modification programme would involve more visits to the clinician, more time, more effort, and more cost. Losing the weight this way would be less attractive than losing it as a result of medication, so let us assign a value of $+70$ to this combination. Not losing weight would obviously be less desirable than not losing it as a result of medication, because of the extra time, effort and costs involved so let us assign this outcome a value of -60. The third treatment is the most demanding of all in terms of effort, costs and time, and also demands regular medical check-ups over a lengthy period. Losing weight this way would, therefore, be much less desirable than losing weight by the other methods, so let us assign a value of $+50$ to this outcome. Even worse would be to go through all the rigours of the combined behaviour modification and very low calorie diet programme and not lose the desired amount of weight, so let us assign a value of -100 to this combination. To make our decision we also need to know the probabilities of losing the desired amount of weight if we undertook a given treatment. From the literature it would seem that the probabilities of losing 9 kg by taking anorectic drugs, undertaking a behaviour modification programme, and adding a very low calorie diet to this are about 0.18, 0.33, and 0.66 respectively (Wing and Jeffery, 1979;

Miller and Sims, 1981; Ley, 1985; Blackburn, Lynch and Wong, 1986). What we do next is weight the values we have already assigned to the outcomes by their probabilities of occurrence, and find the total weighted value for each row. (The technical term for this is an *expected utility*.) This has been done in Figure 10.2. It can be seen that the weighted sum with the highest value (or in this case, the least negative one) is the one associated with the combination of behaviour modification and a very low calorie diet.

It is obviously possible to argue about the weights attached, whether events should have been considered, whether more treatment possibilities should have been considered and so on. There are also other possible decision rules. (For a brief elementary review of behavioural decision theory see Wright (1984).) However, what is important is that the example shows that for the patient or client and, equally importantly, for the clinician to make a rational decision about treatment the following information is needed:

(a) a list of the alternative treatments;
(b) a list of the possible events;
(c) the probabilities of those events occurring with and without treatment;
(d) consideration of the weightings to be attached to each outcome.

Figure 10.2: The hypothetical pay-off matrix for the treatment of obesity problem with utilities, probabilities and expected utilities shown

Treatment choices	Events		Sum of weighted utilities
	Weight lost	Weight not lost	
Medication	$+ 100 \times 0.18$ $= + 18$	$- 50 \times 0.82$ $= - 41$	-23.0
Behaviour modification	$+ 70 \times 0.33$ $= + 23.1$	$- 60 \times 0.67$ $+ - 40.2$	-17.1
Behaviour modification plus very low calorie diet	$+ 50 \times 0.66$ $= + 33$	$- 100 \times 0.33$ $= - 33$	0.0

Obviously no-one expects that patients will start using pay-off matrices in the consulting room (but with the spread of microcomputers who knows?). What is clear though is that for patients to be in a position to make a rational decision they would need information which is probably not normally provided. It is worth noting in passing that Sutton (1982) and Sutton and Eiser (1984) make use of decision theory and expected subjective utilities in their analyses of smoking behaviour and the effects of fear-arousing communications.

GENERATING THE UNIVERSE OF POSSIBLE TOPICS OF INFORMATION

This forbidding sounding procedure is no more than a method for listing all the topics about which patients might be informed. Ley (1978) suggested that it might be possible to generate a series of decision trees which would be generally applicable. These would provide a series of questions to which the clinician or patient would simply have to answer 'yes' or 'no'. From the answers so obtained it would then be clear whick sorts of information should be provided. An example of such a tree concerned with information about indications for use of the drug is shown in Figure 10.3. The basic statement is that the patient's condition is an indication for the use of the drug. The clinician or patient then has to follow the branches of the tree and make decisions at each point until the answer is 'no'. Such

Figure 10.3: A possible tree diagram for deciding what information should be given about the indications for the use of a particular treatment

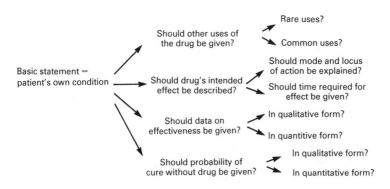

trees can easily be generated for information about the name of the drug, side-effects, contraindications, adverse reactions, interactions with other drugs, dosage, interactions with everyday substances and so on. Once more it is the principle which is important, so do not become too involved in the exact details of this example.

EMPIRICAL CRITERIA

This can be a very brief section. Selection by empirical criteria would mean that we would include in the information given to patients those particular bits of information which have been shown to be associated with the desired outcomes. Thus in the light of the research by Korsch *et al.* (1968) we might decide to include the reasons why certain of the patients' expectations are not to be met, and spend some time talking about non-medical topics if we wished to increase patients' satisfaction. Obviously much of what has been said in previous chapters is relevant here.

MOTIVATIONAL CONTENT

The possible use of the Health Belief Model

The Health Belief Model has already been mentioned several times. It has also been stressed that the model seems to be well supported by the available evidence. It will be recalled that the Model predicts that the probability of an individual adopting a health conducive behaviour is affected by that individual's perceptions of:

(a) their susceptibility to the illness or danger;
(b) the severity or seriousness of that illness or danger;
(c) the effectiveness or benefit of following the recommended course of action;
(d) the material and psychological costs of, and barriers to, the adoption of the behaviour.

As we have seen research has provided strong support for the Model. Table 10.3 is a summary based on the review of studies by Janz and Becker (1984).

In view of these findings, one source of information about what sort of motivating information should be provided is an examination of the patients' Health Beliefs. If they do not

Table 10.3: Summary of findings from Health Belief Model studies

Health Belief Model Variable	Number of studies showing result:		
	Significant in right direction	Not significant	Significant in wrong direction
Vulnerability/susceptibility	30	5	2
Severity	24	12	1
Effectiveness/benefits	29	8	0
Barriers/costs	25	3	0

understand their vulnerability to the condition, its seriousness, or the effectiveness of the recommended actions, then the clinician should provide the necessary information. There have been very few studies which have attempted to influence compliance by systematic application of Health Belief Model concepts. A major investigation which did make such an attempt is that of Inui *et al.* (1976), who showed that the patients of a group of physicians who had had a tutorial on ways of using the Health Belief Model to reduce non-compliance in hypertension had better knowledge of hypertension, better compliance with the medication regimen and better blood pressure control than the patients of doctors who had not had the tutorial. Sixty-nine per cent of the patients whose doctors had had the tutorial showed good blood pressure control, compared with only 36 per cent of the other patients. Unfortunately, as Janz and Becker (1984) point out, the interpretation of these results is complicated by the fact that the tutored physicians received information, not given to the other physicians, about levels of compliance in their patients and, furthermore, no data were collected to show that patients' health beliefs had been changed. Nevertheless this study should encourage future efforts to assess the utility of the model in changing patients' behaviour.

The use of fear appeals and one-sided versus two-sided messages

Research into the effectiveness of fear appeals in persuading people to change their attitudes and behaviour has been an active topic of research for many years (Janis, 1967; Leventhal, 1970; Sutton, 1982). Further, in the case of clinically relevant material, even if no deliberate attempt is made to induce fear the material presented will often be intrinsically likely to arouse fear. As well as a good brief review of the theories in the field Sutton (1982) has provided a meta-analytic study of the effects of fear-arousing communications on attitudes and behaviour. The results of the 38 investigations he summarises give rise to the following conclusions:

(a) fear arousal increases the probability that people will accept recommendations and follow advice;
(b) the danger that material causing higher levels of fear might be counterproductive does not seem to be supported by the evidence;
(c) increasing efficacy of the recommended action increases the probability that it will be adopted;
(d) (less certainly) it seems that the provision of specific instructions about how to perform the recommended action also increases the probability of its being performed.

However, the evidence does not consistently show advantages for fear-arousing communications over neutral communications. Thus Ley *et al.* (1974) and Skilbeck, Tulips, and Ley (1977) did not find that high fear messages led to greater weight loss in obese women. However, Skilbeck *et al.* also investigated the effect of fear *aroused in the subjects* by the message they received. It is clearly sensible to do this because although on average high fear messages will arouse more fear in subjects than low fear messages, there will be a range of reactions to the messages. Thus some of those exposed to a high fear message will not be frightened, whereas some of those exposed to a low fear message will be. Skilbeck *et al.* found that those reacting with medium levels of fear arousal lost more weight than those reacting with low or high fear.

A further experiment on the effects of messages varying in fear level was conducted by Ley, Whitworth, Woodward and Yorke (1977), who sent, on a random basis, one of three letters to all of the obese patients in a British general practice. The letters varied in judged level of fear-arousing potential, and it was found that variation in this had no effect on the numbers expressing a wish for further information, nor on the numbers willing to join a slimming programme.

Other recent studies report mixed findings. Glanz, Kirscht

and Rosenstock (1981) found no effect of level of fear arousal in a printed message given to hypertensive patients, but Sutton and Eiser (1984) found that a fear-arousing film about smoking caused more smokers to express the intention of trying to quit than did a control film. Unfortunately the control film was not about smoking so it is unclear as to whether it was the fear-arousing nature of the film or its informational content which caused the effect.

Skilbeck *et al.* (1977) also investigated the effects of the position of the fear appeal, and the effects of single versus multiple exposures to the message. Weight loss was significantly greater when the fear-arousing message was placed just before the recommendations, than when there was intervening text between it and the recommendations, than when it followed the recommendations. This investigation also found that those exposed once only to the fear-arousing message lost more weight than those given multiple reminders of it. Other investigators have reported a variety of findings concerning the effects of repeated exposure to messages. Horowitz (1969) gave subjects one or five presentations of a message concerning drug abuse. There were no differences in attitude between those receiving the different numbers of exposures. On the other hand Kirscht and Haefner (1973) reported that subjects exposed to one, two or three screenings of a film on heart disease showed differential behavioural and attitudinal reactions. In general more exposures led to more change, but there were some interactions in the study which make this summary a little over-simplified. Thus the Kirscht and Haefner investigation shows an effect of repetition up to three repetitions; Horowitz using five repetitions obtained no effect and Skilbeck *et al.* found 50-plus repetitions to be less effective than a single exposure. This was true for all of the three different levels of fear arousal used. The results obtained by Skilbeck *et al.* are shown in Figure 10.4.

This collection of findings clearly suggests the possibility that the relationship between number of repetitions and effectiveness of the message is curvilinear. This suggestion receives some support from two experiments reported by Cacioppo and Petty (1979). These investigators studied the effects of one, three and five exposures to a message and found in both experiments that agreement with the message was higher for three exposures than for one or five. Unfortunately the message was not a health-related message.

Figure 10.4: Differences in weight loss, over a 16-week period, for three samples of subjects given single or multiple exposures to a fear-arousing message

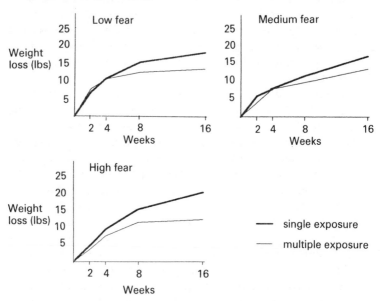

To sum up, fear-arousal seems to increase the probability of change in attitudes and behaviour, but it does not always do so. Its effectiveness probably depends on the specificity of the recommended actions and on the perceived effectiveness of those actions in averting the danger referred to in the message. Its effectiveness also varies with its position in the message and on with the number of times the individual is exposed to it. There is very little evidence that fear-arousing messages produce worse results than neutral messages, despite the well-known early findings of Janis and Feshbach (1953).

Ley *et al.* (1974, 1979) and Skilbeck *et al.* (1977) also investigated the effects of using two-sided as opposed to one-sided messages. In brief, one-sided messages just present one side of the argument, while two-sided messages discuss both sides of the question, going into both the pros and the cons of the advocated position. The usual summary of research into their effects with non-health-related materials is that one-sided messages probably produce most change in situations where the individual is not likely to be exposed to counterarguments, but that two-sided presentations produce greater long-term change if later exposure to counterarguments occurs. In the series of experiments conducted by these investigators it was found that there were no differences in weight loss between obese women exposed to one-sided or two-sided presentations, but that this variable did affect desire for more information about, and willingness to volunteer for a slimming programme among unselected obese patients. The percentages (a) wanting more information and (b) wishing to participate in the slimming programme were, for those receiving the two-sided presentation, 68 and 68 per cent respectively, while for those receiving the one-sided presentation they were 54 and 43 per cent. The findings need to be replicated in other situations and other conditions.

MALIGNANT COMPLIANCE

Having claimed that fear arousal can often be a strong per-suasive force it might be just as well to include a cautionary tale.

Malignant compliance is a concept introduced by Norell (1982b) in a letter to *The Lancet*. While this may be an unfor-tunate form of words, smacking as it does of damning the patient for too much as well as too little compliance, the intended point is an important one. In his letter he described the case of a female 63-year-old patient with glaucoma for whom pilocarpine eye drops had been prescribed. She had been told to use her drops at 7 a.m., 2 p.m. and 9 p.m., and had been using the drops for four years or so before she became involved in a study of medication compliance using Norell's medication monitor, a device for the automatic recording of the time when a medication container is used. Examination of a 40 day record showed only one deviation from the prescribed time for taking the medicine. On one occasion she had been one hour late with her 9 p.m. dose. Because such levels of accuracy in medicine taking are very rarely seen she was interviewed about this. It transpired that she had been in a permanent state of anxiety and fear that she would lose her sight if she did not comply precisely with the instructions. Her doctor had told her that she would go blind if she did not use the drops *exactly* as directed. This was a remarkably successful use of fear arousal from the point of view of compliance, but it was clearly achieved at an undesirable cost. Obviously the doctor had not intended that the patient should think that the timing had to be exactly accurate on all occasions. But lack of understanding combined with fear

155

arousal had meant a very anxious four years for this patient.

SUMMARY

This chapter has outlined some of the criteria for deciding on the content of the information to be presented to patients. The possible criteria include:

(a) patients' opinions;
(b) professionals' opinions;
(c) behaviourally defined objectives;
(d) what is needed for rational decision making;
(e) judgemental criteria;
(f) empirical criteria.

These criteria can be used to select the topics of information to be given to patients.

It is likely that the persuasive and motivational impact of the message can be improved by using the Health Belief Model to discover the areas where patients' beliefs militate against acceptance of the message. Unfortunately there seems to have been little research on this topic. However, there is at least one study reporting encouraging results, and in other respects the basic tenets of the Model seem to be well supported by research results.

The use of fear-arousing communications also seems likely to lead to greater acceptance of recommendations. Its effectiveness will depend on a variety of factors which probably include the following:

(a) how specific the recommendations are;
(b) whether they are seen as effective ways of averting the threatened danger;
(c) the frequency with which the individual is exposed to the message — it seems possible that a message can be repeated too many times;
(d) the position of the fear-arousing content in relation to the recommendations — probably immediately before the recommendations is best;
(e) there are very mixed findings on the relative merits of one-sided and two-sided messages.

Because there has been little research on some of these points the findings should be regarded as very tentative.

11

The Benefits of Improved Communication

INTRODUCTION

This chapter will consider the question of the extent to which improved communication is likely to achieve the aims required of it. These aims include at least the following:

(a) increased patient knowledge and recall;
(b) increased patient satisfaction;
(c) genuinely informed consent;
(d) increased patient compliance;
(e) quicker recovery from illness.

Each of these will now be considered.

INCREASED PATIENT KNOWLEDGE AND RECALL

There has already been so much discussion of patients' knowledge and recall that this section can be a brief one. It has been shown that patients' understanding and recall can be improved by a variety of techniques. Summaries of the effectiveness of these methods have been given in Chapters 6 and 9. Use of primacy effects, stressed importance, simplification, explicit categorisation, specific statements, and repetition increase patients' recall and understanding of their condition, and the techniques can be effectively used by general practitioners (Ley, *et al.*, 1976b). Providing physicians with brief teaching about the Health Belief Model also seems capable of changing their behaviour in ways that enhance their patients' understanding

(Inui, Yourtee and Williamson, 1976). In addition to these experimental studies there is ample correlational evidence to show that provision of information is associated with patients' understanding, e.g. Smith *et al.* (1981).

As would be expected the provision of written information also seems reliably to increase patients' knowledge. Thus Ley and Morris (1984) found that written information had been found to increase patients' knowledge in 97 per cent of the studies they reviewed. However, it will be recalled that written information is frequently pitched at too hard a level for its intended audience.

The techniques of meta-analysis have also been applied to the problem of the effectiveness of improved communication in increasing patients' knowledge and understanding. It will be recalled that meta-analysis allows reviewers to aggregate, in a quantitative fashion, the results of studies using a variety of different methods. This is done by converting the result of each study into an 'effect size', which is a standardised index, which can be compared across studies. The two commonest measures of effect size have been:

(a) the difference between treatment and control means divided by the standard deviation of the control group, e.g. Smith, Glass and Miller (1980);
(b) the correlation coefficient between the treatment variable and the outcome measure, e.g. Shoham-Salomon and Rosenthal (1987).

Other techniques are also used, but whatever the technique, the higher the effect size the stronger is the treatment effect.

Mullen, Green and Persinger (1985) have provided a meta-analysis of clinical trials of attempts to improve patients' knowledge by a variety of methods likely to improve the communication of information. The methods included the provision of additional face to face consultation, group education, written information, and combinations of some of these. The mean effect size for the data reported by these reviewers was +0.53. This can be interpreted as showing that the average patient who received these additional educational inputs had better knowledge and understanding than 70 per cent of those who had not received this extra input.

Thus, as would be expected, time spent in providing information to patients seems to increase their knowledge and understanding of their condition. Further, understanding and recall can be enhanced by the use of special techniques and by the provision of suitably prepared written or audiovisual materials.

INCREASED PATIENT SATISFACTION

Earlier in this book the evidence that people seem to want to know as much as possible about their condition, its treatment, its prognosis, and its aetiology has been presented. In view of this it is hardly surprising that there is plenty of experimental and correlational evidence to show that informed patients are more satisfied. The correlational evidence has been presented in some detail in Chapter 5. Experimental studies have, for example, shown that taking steps to increase patients' understanding of what they have been told increases their levels of satisfaction (Ley, *et al.*, 1976a), and that improving recall of what has been said also increases patients' satisfaction (Bertakis, 1977). Other findings suggest ways of improving patients' satisfaction by ensuring that the clinician attempts to find out what the patients' expectations are, and that all of the patients' worries have been aired (Korsch *et al.*, 1968).

Thus it would seem that the first two aims of improved communication are often achieved.

GENUINELY INFORMED CONSENT

The main problem here lies in the definition of 'genuinely informed consent' (President's Commission for the Study of Ethical Problems in Medicine and Biomedical and Behavioral Research, 1982; Faden, Beauchamp and King, 1986). It is easy enough to indicate situations where it does not exist, e.g. when patients are presented with a written consent form that they do not understand — a situation which, as we have seen, is probably all too common (e.g. Morrow 1980). Clearly then a minimal requirement for informed consent is that the material presented to the patient should be understandable. Further it should also be rememberable so that patients can reconsider it if they wish.

This still leaves lots of problems about the content of

informed consent messages. Again as a minimum they should contain information about:

(a) the benefits and risks of the proposed treatment and their probabilities of occurrence;
(b) the benefits and risks of alternative treatments and their probabilities of occurrence;
(c) the probabilities of the various outcomes if the patient decided to have no treatment at all.

As we have seen the communication of risk information is desired by patients and it does not seem to have the adverse effects that clinicians sometimes fear it will have (e.g. Alfidi, 1970).

The question of how best to present risk probabilities to people is still unresolved, and it is known that different ways of presenting the same information can make a big difference to people's choices. A good example of this is the problem that Tversky and Kahneman (1981) put to a sample of physicians. Suppose that the country is preparing for the outbreak of an unusual disease, which is expected to kill 600 people. Two alternative programmes are available to fight the disease. If the first programme (A) is adopted 200 people will be saved. If the second programme (B) is adopted there is a one-third probability that 600 people will be saved and a two-thirds probability that no people will be saved. Which of the two programmes do you prefer?

Suppose further that there is a third programme (C) which, if adopted, will lead to 400 people dying, and a fourth programme (D), which gives a one-third probability that nobody will die and a two-thirds probability that 600 people will die. Which of programmes C and D do you prefer?

In Tversky and Kahneman's study 75 per cent of physicians chose programme A over programme B, and 67 per cent chose programme D over programme C. But of course on close examination A and C are identical options as are B and D. Thus it can be seen that even health professionals can be much affected by the way in which probability information is presented.

In another clinically relevant study Fischoff, Slovic and Lichtenstein (1981) asked people to estimate the chances of dying from a variety of diseases such as diabetes, hypertension,

asthma, strokes and cancer. For hypertension the questions and
the corresponding estimates were as follows:

Question	Estimated deaths per 100 000
For every 100 000 people with high blood pressure how many will die from it?	535
X people have high blood pressure, how many will die from it?	89
For every person who dies from high blood pressure how many survive?	17
If Y people have died from high blood pressure, how many will suffer from it but survive?	538

It can be seen that the wording of the question can have a
large effect on the estimated risk. Similarly, McNeil, Pauker,
Sox and Tversky (1982) studied samples of (a) patients, (b)
physicians, and (c) graduate students, who were provided with
data on the survival rates of patients with lung cancer treated by
surgery or by radiation. The subjects had to make judgements
about which treatment was the more acceptable. Judgements
were strongly affected by whether the data were presented in
terms of chances of dying or chances of survival. In the first case
42 per cent would prefer radiation, in the second case only 25
per cent would. This effect was noticed in all three groups of
subjects.

Stanley, Guido, Stanley and Shortell (1984) investigated the
ability of patients to make sensible decisions on the basis of
information provided about risks and benefits. Patients'
performance was measured on three dimensions:

(a) comprehension of the material;
(b) quality of reasoning about the decision made;
(c) the reasonableness of the choices made.

It was found that the choices of both older and younger patients
were appropriately affected by the relative risks and benefits,
but that older patients had greater difficulty in understanding
the information provided, and showed poorer quality reasoning
in reaching their decision.

Finally with regard to risk information it would appear that the words used to represent the outcome will affect people's perceptions of the dangers involved. Thus, Keown, cited by Slovic, Fischoff and Lichtenstein (1980) found that 'abnormal bruising' as a side-effect of medication caused much more concern that 'a tendency to develop black and blue marks'.

For further discussion of the still-unresolved problems of presenting risk information and probability information generally see Schwartz (1979), Slovic et al. (1980), Fischoff, Lichtenstein, Slovic, Derby and Keeney (1981), Eraker and Politser (1982) and Kahneman, Slovic and Tversky (1982).

Having pointed out these problems and having failed to specify exactly what 'genuine informed consent' is it is nevertheless clear that improved communication will reduce the frequency of ill-informed consent.

INCREASED PATIENT COMPLIANCE

Meta-analytic techniques have been applied to the problem of the effectiveness of communication-improving techniques on patients' compliance. These studies have often also provided data on the effectiveness of behaviour-modification techniques. The behavioural techniques are similar to the behavioural techniques used generally in clinical work for the alleviation of patients' disorders, and have included the following:

(a) stimulus control, by increasing the salience of the cues associated with medicine taking, or by 'tailoring' the regimen to the patient's routine and events therein;

(b) self-monitoring of medication use, and/or symptoms, and/or dosage;

(c) reinforcement of compliance or outcome by the use of positive and negative reinforcement, contracts, response cost procedures, and drug level feedback;

(d) programmed learning;

(e) prompting by alarms and reminders.

The reader interested in these techniques can find fuller details in DiMatteo and DiNicola (1982), Epstein and Cluss (1982), Cameron and Best (1987) and Meichenbaum and Turk (1987). As will be seen there is good evidence for their effectiveness in reducing non-compliance.

The next few paragraphs will contain many estimates of percentages compliant. As compliance rates vary according to a variety of factors the figures discussed are average ones and the reader should, therefore, regard the reported estimates as subject to error. In addition some of the techniques used for deriving some of the estimates are relatively novel and might be open to later objection. A final point is that many of the interventions used in attempts to increase patients' knowledge and compliance have involved the use of written information. As we have seen earlier, much of the written information provided to patients is sub-optimal in a variety of ways. This probably means that the results of such interventions might perhaps be better regarded as minimum rather than maximum estimates.

Mazzuca (1982) reported a meta-analyis of what he classified as didactic and behavioural patient education. The didactic category included studies which used lectures, pamphlets, audiovisual media, and prescription labels in an attempt to present standard information about the condition and its treatment to all patients with that condition. Mazzuca's behavioural category included studies which tried to individualise instruction for patients and fit regimens into their individual daily routines, and studies using some of the techniques listed earlier. The mean effect sizes were, for didactic techniques +0.26, and for behavioural techniques, +0.64. Thus it would be expected that the average patient exposed to didactic techniques would be more compliant than 60 per cent, and the average patient receiving behavioural instruction than 73 per cent of those given no such instruction.

The meta-analysis of Mullen *et al.* (1985) also presented an effect size for the effects of instructional and educational methods on compliance. Studies were not categorised in the same way as in Mazzuca's analysis, but reported an overall effect size for compliance as measured by drug errors of +0.37, with the category 'Behavior modification/self administration' yielding an effect size of +0.50. These figures can be interpreted as showing that the average patient exposed to such interventions is more compliant than 64 per cent (overall result) and 69 per cent (behaviour modification) of patients receiving no intervention.

A further way of interpreting the results of meta-analyses where a baseline value is known has been suggested by Ley (1987b). If we take the weighted mean of the medication compliance studies reported by the Department of Health, Education and Welfare (1979) as a base this gives us an expected compliance rate of 52 per cent without any intervention. Using Ley's method it would be estimated that the use of Mazzuca's didactic interventions, and the techniques summarised by Mullen *et al.* would increase the percentage compliant to 62 and 66 per cent respectively. For behavioural techniques the corresponding figures would be 75 and 71 per cent. These estimates are consistent with the average figure of a 23 per cent increase in compliance given in the conventional narrative review of behavioural methods for increasing compliance (Haynes, 1982), which, given a base of 52 per cent compliant, would suggest that the use of behavioural techniques would lead to 75 per cent being compliant.

Ley (1986a) used a different approach to this problem arguing that the Behavioral Effect Size Display (BESD) technique proposed by Rosenthal and Rubin (1982) could be applied. This technique enables one to derive percentages in different outcome categories from a given correlation coefficient. Figure 11.1 shows the correlations between the variables in the cognitive model and compliance.

Using the BESD method it would be estimated that 68 per cent of patients with adequate understanding, and 63 per cent of patients with adequate levels of satisfaction would be compliant. The corresponding figures for patients without such levels of understanding and satisfaction would be 32 and 37 per cent.

Figure 11.1: Summary of the mean correlations between understanding, memory, satisfaction and compliance

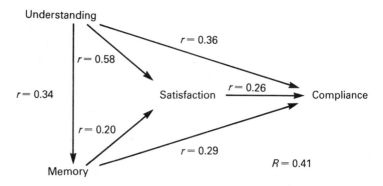

The conclusions from these studies would seem to be that both didactic and behavioural approaches can lead to improvement in compliance, but that the behavioural approach leads to greater gains. Unfortunately behavioural methods tend to be expensive compared with, say, the use of supplementary written information. Certainly they are too expensive for general use in all cases where compliance might be a problem. Supplementary written information on the other hand is relatively cheap, and its use could well lead to significant savings on health care. For example, Ley (1986a) calculated that if the use of supplementary written information increased compliance rates to 66 per cent, then in 1979 dollars there would be a saving in the USA of 114–228 million US dollars just for the ten drugs reviewed by the Department of Health, Education and Welfare (1979).

There are also some further complications in the interpretation of studies on the comparative effectiveness of informational and other intervention strategies. Ley (1979b) has argued that non-compliant behaviours can be classified along two dimensions. The first is whether the non-complier is adequately informed or not. The second is whether the non-compliance is intentional or unintentional. This classification yields the four cells shown in Figure 11.2.

The adequately informed intentional non-complier is clearly not likely to be affected by simple educational/informative input. This person already knows the nature of the illness, its

Figure 11.2: The different types of non-compliance and the intervention techniques likely to affect them

LEVEL OF KNOWLEDGE

	Adequate	Inadequate
Intentional	Persuasion	More information
Unintentional	Memory aids	More information

risks, the effectiveness of treatment and so on, yet despite this has decided not to comply with the recommended regimen. The inadequately informed intentional non-complier is perhaps well exemplified by the people in the study of Spelman and Ley (1966) who, although they knew that lung cancer was caused by smoking, thought that it was easily curable. Such people might well become compliant with advice about trying to quit smoking if properly informed about the prognosis of lung cancer. Note of course that the information could also have the effect of merely making them adequately informed non-compliers. The main reason for adequately informed unintentional non-compliance is simply forgetting to take the tablet or follow the regimen at the appropriate time or place. Information provision would not be expected to have any effect here. The last category consists of non-compliance where the patient thinks that they are in fact complying, but because of misunderstanding the instructions is not in fact doing so. A patient who had been instructed to take the tablets four times a day and took all four at once after breakfast would fall into this category. It would be expected that non-compliance of this sort would be affected by the provision of correct information. The effectiveness of the provision of information (in suitable form) in reducing non-compliance will thus depend on the type of non-compliance involved. In comparative studies it will depend on the relative proportions of patients in the different categories. Both inadequate information and intentional non-compliance can be quite frequent. Thus, Parkin *et al.* (1976) found that 70 per cent of their non-compliant patients had inadequate knowledge of the regimen, and Cooper *et al.* (1982) reported that 73 per cent of their non-compliant patients were intentional non-compliers. Unfortunately there seem to be no studies which report on the proportions of patients falling into each of the four cells. These would of course be expected to vary from illness to illness and regimen to regimen, and to be affected by patient characteristics.

EFFECTS OF IMPROVED COMMUNICATION ON RECOVERY FROM ILLNESS AND SURGERY

There are now many investigations of the effects of enhanced communication on recovery of surgical patients and on reactions to invasive investigative and dental procedures. Ley (1977) classified these interventions as (a) information giving — the patient is given an account of what is going to happen and when it is going to happen; (b) instruction — the patient is given information on what to do to reduce pain and discomfort, e.g. how to cough, how to turn in bed, how to use a trapeze; and (c) quasi-therapeutic — the patient is given the opportunity to air fears, discuss worries and receive reassurance. It is highly probable that in real life these procedures are seldom used alone. It is likely that most communication-enhancing interventions use elements of all of them. In a review of 13 studies which had explored the effects of these procedures on recovery from surgery Ley concluded that there seemed to be a reduction in length of hospitalisation, and in need for analgesics in patients receiving such enhanced communication. However, there were methodological problems with most of the investigations, notably the lack of placebo control groups, so any conclusions had to be tentative.

Anderson and Masur (1983) also reviewed the literature but used a rather different classification system to categorise the interventions they reviewed. They divided these into (a) informative approaches, (b) psychotherapeutic approaches, (c) modelling, (d) behavioural approaches, (e) cognitive behavioural approaches and (f) hypnotic approaches. The main forms of informative information studied were procedural information and sensation information. Procedural information consists of a description of what will happen and when it will happen. Sensation information tells the patient what sensations can be expected at various stages in the procedure and in recovery. This distinction was important in the light of research and theorising by Johnson and Leventhal (1974), Johnson (1975), Johnson, Fuller, Endress and Rice (1978) and Leventhal, Brown, Shacham and Engquist (1979) suggesting a special role for sensation information. In the modelling procedures the patient sees a film or video of someone going through the procedures. This model sometimes shows little anxiety or sometimes shows anxiety and is then shown coping with it in various ways. Most research into modelling has been concerned with preparing children for hospital. In the behavioural technique category Anderson and Masur included training in relaxation as well as more complicated techniques such as systematic desensitisation, but also included what Ley had termed instruction, e.g.

how to cough, how to swallow during endoscopic investigations and so on. Cognitive-behavioural approaches are based on the assumption that the patient's cognitions about surgery or other invasive procedures will have a major effect on the stress felt by the patient. If maladaptive cognitions can be identified and modified then the patient's adjustment to the stresses involved should be improved.

Noting that the area was still plagued by methodological problems, Anderson and Masur concluded:

(a) pre-operative information alone can probably have beneficial effects on outcome;
(b) the best results seem to be obtained by using a combination of sensation and procedural information;
(c) the value of brief psychotherapy as a preparatory strategy remains to be demonstrated;
(d) the use of modelling procedures has produced beneficial results;
(e) behavioural techniques seem to help reduce anxiety and fear;
(f) research into the use of cognitive-behavioural techniques suggests that they also are of use;
(g) because of severe methodological problems the usefulness of hypnosis has yet to be demonstrated, but many clinicians consider it to be valuable.

The conclusions of most interest in the present context are those suggesting that enhanced information provision can have beneficial effects.

A further review was presented by Mathews and Ridgeway (1984). This time pre-operative preparation techniques were classified as (a) procedural information, (b) sensation information, (c) behavioural instructions, e.g. how to cough, (d) modelling, (e) relaxation and (f) cognitive coping training. This last category was very similar to the cognitive–behavioural category of Anderson and Masur. Mathews and Ridgeway were particularly concerned with the results of studies they considered to be methodologically sound, but found very few of these. Their conclusions included the following:

(a) information and behavioural instruction can form an effective component of preparation, especially if the information provided includes adequate descriptions of the sensations to be experienced;

(b) training in cognitive coping strategies appears to be beneficial;

(c) patients with high anxiety seem to benefit more than less anxious patients from preparatory communications.

In addition to these narrative reviews there have been meta-analytic studies of educational and instructional interventions on recovery from surgery, the progress of illness and its outcome. Mazzuca (1982) reported that the mean effect sizes for didactic methods on progress and outcome were +0.18, and +0.19 respectively, suggesting that the average patient exposed to these interventions would be better off than about 57 per cent of those not treated in this way. Behaviourally oriented methods were better, producing effect sizes of +0.74 for progress, and +0.31 for outcome.

Mumford, Schlesinger and Glass (1982) also performed a meta-analysis. Interventions included most of those already described. The studies analysed were concerned with recovery from surgery and heart attack. The mean effect size for these interventions was +0.43. Educational approaches produced a mean effect size of +0.30. Thus the average patient receiving an educational intervention would be expected to progress better than 61 per cent of those not receiving this intervention. These reviewers also reported that patients receiving interventions needed to remain about two days less in hospital. However, the mean difference between those receiving an informational intervention and their controls was a little less, being only 1.21 days.

Another meta-analysis using a sample of 49 investigations was reported by Devine and Cook (1983). This meta-analysis confirmed that psycho-educational interventions reduced patient stay in hospital. On average, stay was reduced by 1.31 days. Devine and Cook also found that the more recent studies yielded a lower estimate of reduction in length of stay. This might be because the value of psycho-educational intervention is now so well accepted that it has become part of the usual routine, or it might be due to the more analytic nature of the more recent studies, which have been trying to tease out the effects of different components in such interventions. This has inevitably led to quite narrow and highly circumscribed interventions being used in the different experimental groups, e.g.

only information provision or *only* instruction or *only* quasi-therapeutic intervention. Devine and Cook suggest that the best results are obtained with intervention packages which include two or three of these components.

Taken overall the results reviewed above suggest that improved information giving reduces distress and speeds up recovery. In view of the cost of a patient day in hospital, and the relative cheapness of informational interventions they are almost certainly highly cost effective.

SUMMARY

This chapter has tried to assess whether the expected benefits of improved communication actually occur. These expected benefits are:

(a) increased patient understanding and recall;
(b) increased patient satisfaction;
(c) less ill-informed consent;
(d) increased patient compliance;
(e) quicker and less stressful recovery from illness and surgery.

Improving communication by either increasing the amount of information provided or by using special techniques can often lead to increased understanding, recall, and satisfaction. Further, because much of the informed consent information presented to patients is probably too difficult for most of them, the chances of reducing ill-informed consent can also be enhanced by simplification of material, and by the use of the other techniques for improving understanding and recall.

It also seems likely that the provision of more information in a better packaged form can help reduce the chances of non-compliance. Better results can be obtained by the use of behavioural techniques, but in many situations their cost would be too high for their use to be justified. The use of properly prepared written information or more careful verbal counselling of patients, although less effective than the behavioural methods, might be cost-effective in many situations.

Finally, it has been shown that improved communication in the form of information (especially sensation information) and/

or behavioural instruction, and/or quasi-psychotherapeutic methods (especially of the behavioural sort) can significantly reduce hospital stay, and make for less-stressful surgical and investigative procedures.

12

A Summary and Some Practical Conclusions

INTRODUCTION

It is now time to summarise the findings of the previous chapters. It will be obvious from what has been said earlier that many of the summary statements which follow should be treated as interim rather than final conclusions. Because the qualifications attached to these conclusions have already been spelt out in some detail in the appropriate chapters they will not be repeated here. But the reader should bear in mind that in some cases the qualifications were major ones.

After the summary statements there is some practical advice about how communications might be improved. This is accompanied by a diagrammatic checklist, which, it is hoped will serve as a convenient reminder of some of the major factors to be considered in better communication with patients.

SATISFACTION WITH COMMUNICATIONS

The main findings about satisfaction with communications are as follows.

(a) Satisfaction with the communications aspect of the consultation correlates highly with satisfaction with other aspects of the clinician–patient interaction.

(b) Substantial numbers of patients feel dissatisfied with the communications aspect of their clinical encounters. This contrasts with usually high levels of satisfaction with other aspects of the clinician–patient interaction.

(c) This dissatisfaction does not seem to be reduced by clinicians trying (in untutored ways) to see that patients are fully informed.

(d) The increase in educational and research concern with the problem, which has taken place over the last two decades, does not seem to have led to a reduction in levels of patients' dissatisfaction.

(e) In addition there is evidence that patients who say that they have been told about various aspects of their condition are just as likely to be dissatisfied as those who say they have not.

(f) Thus it is clear that telling patients is in itself not enough. They have to be told in ways that they can understand and remember, and attempts have to be made to ascertain what the patient's informational needs are.

(g) Because of lack of feedback from patients in the form of questions and comments it is difficult for clinicians to improve their performance as communicators.

UNDERSTANDING

Investigations of patients' understanding of what they have been told have shown:

(a) Patients often do not know the meanings of the words used by the clinician.

(b) Patients often have their own ideas about illnesses and these often differ from the accepted orthodox ideas.

(c) What the clinician says will be interpreted in terms of the patient's own framework of ideas.

(d) As measured by the patient's own report, or by expert judgement, or by quasi-behavioural tests, patients often fail to understand what they are told by health care professionals.

(e) Patients are often reluctant to ask for further information even when they would very much like it.

MEMORY

The findings reviewed can be summarised as follows.

(a) Patients often forget a great deal of what they are told.
(b) The time elapsing between presentation and recall of the material has virtually no relation to how much is recalled.
(c) In studies of hospital outpatients and in analogue studies the number of statements presented is linearly related to mean percentage recalled.
(d) In studies of general practice patients this relationship is not apparent.
(e) There appears to be no consistent relationship between the age of the patient and the amount recalled. There is, however, some suggestion that patients over age 65 perhaps have poorer recall.
(f) The patient's intellectual and educational level have only a low relationship to recall.
(g) The individual's general level of medical knowledge is related to recall.
(h) Anxiety is related to recall. The lower the anxiety the worse the recall.
(i) There appears to be a primacy effect in recall of medical information. People recall best what they are told first.
(j) Statements that seem important to patients are more likely to be recalled.

IMPROVING UNDERSTANDING AND MEMORY

The results reviewed can be summarised as follows.

(a) Recall of the content of orally presented communications can be increased by the use of:
    (1) primacy effects;
    (2) stressing the importance of particular content.
(b) The amount recalled can be increased by the use of:
    (1) simplification;
    (2) explicit categorisation;
    (3) repetition;
    (4) use of specific rather than general statements;
    (5) mixtures of the above.
(c) Telephoned and mailed reminders are effective in reducing the frequency with which appointments are broken.
(d) A variety of mechanical aids to memory have been tried, mainly with elderly patients and mainly without success.

(e) Simplification improves understanding.
(f) The provision of written back-up materials improves understanding and memory.

WRITTEN INFORMATION

The findings about the use of written information can be summarised as follows.

(a) Its use increases patients' knowledge.
(b) Its use sometimes increases compliance.
(c) It is not always read.
(d) It is frequently too difficult for patients to understand.
(e) Its contents are often forgotten.

THE IMPROVEMENT OF WRITTEN INFORMATION

The disappointingly meagre findings reviewed can be summarised as follows.

(a) Increasing the readability of written information by using shorter words and shorter sentences leads to:
    (1) better understanding;
    (2) better recall;
    (3) sometimes better compliance.
(b) Altering aspects of written material, such as the following, has not, to date, been shown to be effective in improving its usefulness:
    (1) use of the active rather than passive voice;
    (2) avoidance of negative sentences;
    (3) use of imperative rather than prescriptive forms.
(c) The use of illustrations has had no consistent effects.
(d) The use of cartoons has had no effects.

NON-COMPLIANCE BY PATIENTS

The findings about the problem of patients' non-compliance with advice can be summarised as follows.

175

(a) The different methods for assessing compliance are significantly inter-correlated but these inter-correlations are
often low in magnitude.

(b) The most popular method, patients' reports, correlates
significantly with other methods of measurement.

(c) The two methods of assessing compliance which seem to
be most problematical are the use of therapeutic
outcome as a measure and the use of the clinician's guess
as to whether the patient is complying or not.

(d) Different methods of measurement tend to produce
different estimates of the frequency of non-compliance,
which is usually judged lowest by patients' report, somewhat higher by pill counts, and higher still by blood and
urine tests.

(e) As assessed by various mixtures of these measures the
average percentage of patients likely to be non-compliant seems to be between 40 and 50 per cent, but the
range of percentages non-compliant is considerable.

(f) Non-compliance costs a great deal of money.

(g) Non-compliance with medication regimens is a significant
cause of hospital admission.

(h) Factors shown to be associated with non-compliance
include:
(1) patient satisfaction;
(2) understanding;
(3) forgetting;
(4) Health Belief Model variables;
(5) the meeting of patients' expectations;
(6) the duration of the regimen;
(7) the complexity of the regimen;
(8) the level of supervision provided;
(9) the influence of family and friends.

NON-COMPLIANCE BY HEALTH CARE PROFESSIONALS

Just as patients often do not comply with the advice they are
given, so also do health professionals often fail to comply with
official recommendations for optimal patient care. Findings in
this area can be summarised as follows.

(a) Non-compliance by health-care professionals seems to

be surprisingly common.
(b) Factors involved in this non-compliance include:
  (1) lack of knowledge;
  (2) failures of memory;
  (3) low job satisfaction;
  (4) susceptibility to social pressures.
(c) There is some preliminary evidence that professional non-compliance can be reduced by:
  (1) educational efforts;
  (2) reminders;
  (3) behavioural strategies.

SELECTING THE CONTENT OF COMMUNICATIONS

(a) The criteria for deciding on the content of the information to be presented to patients include:
  (1) patients' opinions;
  (2) professionals' opinions;
  (3) behaviourally defined objectives;
  (4) what is needed for rational decision making;
  (5) judgemental criteria;
  (6) empirical criteria.
(b) It is likely that the persuasive and motivational impact of the message can be improved by using the Health Belief Model to discover the areas where patients' beliefs militate against acceptance of the message;
(c) The use of fear-arousing communications also seems likely to lead to greater acceptance of recommendations. Its effectiveness will depend on a variety of factors which tentatively include the following:
  (1) how specific the recommendations are;
  (2) whether they are seen as effective ways of averting the threatened danger;
  (3) the frequency with which the individual is exposed to the message — fewer exposures lead to better results;
  (4) the position of the fear-arousing content in relation to the recommendations.
(d) Two-sided messages sometimes increase the effectiveness of persuasive health communications.

THE BENEFITS OF IMPROVED COMMUNICATIONS

The probable benefits of improving communication in the ways advocated include the following.

(a) Patients' understanding and recall are increased.
(b) Patients are more satisfied.
(c) There is less ill-informed consent.
(d) Compliance is likely to be increased.
(e) Recovery from illness and surgery may be quicker and less stressful.

A BRIEF PRACTICAL GUIDE TO BETTER COMMUNICATION

This section will attempt to provide some practical guidelines for improving communication with patients and clients. The suggestions to be made will cover the following topics:

(a) increasing satisfaction;
(b) selecting the content of the communication;
(c) increasing understanding and recall.

All of these suggestions are of course based on the research reviewed in earlier chapters and summarised above.

Increasing satisfaction

Before even seeing the patient it is possible to reduce the chances of dissatisfaction by having a good appointments system which ensures that patients' waiting time is minimised. If hold-ups and delays are going to occur make sure that those who are waiting know why there is a delay and how long it is likely to be. Long waiting times are associated with low patient satisfaction, and poorer compliance.

Be friendly rather than businesslike, and spend at least some time in conversation about non-clinical topics. Allow patients to tell their story in their own words. Find out what the main worries and what the expectations are. If these expectations are not going to be met explain why this is so. Give plenty of information and explanation.

178

Selecting the content of the communication

Find out what the patient wants to know. Find out what the patient's Health Beliefs are. Does the patient see themselves as vulnerable to the consequences of not following advice? Are those consequences seen as serious? Is the advice seen as being effective in averting those consequences? Do the costs and barriers associated with following the advice seem to be too great? Provide information to correct these perceptions where they are wrong.

Decide what information you want the patient to have. Use a checklist if possible to ensure that nothing important is left out.

Consider the value of fear arousal, but remember the possibly counter-productive effects of too many exposures to a fear message. In many cases the extra effort of presenting a two-sided message will be worthwhile.

Increasing understanding and recall

Avoid jargon and unexplained technical terms. Use short words and short sentences. Encourage feedback by asking the patient if what has been said has been understood. Ask if the patient would like more information.

Use of primacy effects and stressing the importance of particular content will increase the chances of particular parts of the message being recalled. The overall amount recalled can be increased by the use of simplification, explicit categorisation, repetition, and the use of specific rather than general instruction statements.

Where possible provide written back-up. Make sure that this is of acceptable readability by using a readability formula. Make sure that print size is adequate, especially for elderly patients. It is probable that attractive physical packaging, e.g. good quality paper and the use of some colour will increase the chances of the written material being read and kept.

Diagrammatic summary

These suggestions are summarised in Figure 12.1.

179

Figure 12.1: Summary of suggestions for improving communication with patients

SATISFACTION	Short waiting time Be friendly rather than business-like Some talk about non-medical topics Listen to patient Find out what worries are Find out what expectations are — if not to be met say why

SELECTING CONTENT	What does patient want to know
	What are the patient's Health Beliefs:
	     Vulnerability
	     Seriousness
	     Effectiveness
	     Costs and barriers
	What do you want the patient to know
	Would motivating communication help:
	     Fear arousal
	     Sidedness

UNDERSTANDING AND MEMORY	Avoid jargon
	Use short words and short sentences
	     — simplification
	Encourage feedback
	Increase recall
	     Primacy
	     Stressed importance
	     Explicit categorisation
	     Specific rather than general
	     Repetition
	Written back-up
	     readability
	     physical format:
	          letter size
	          colour
	          quality of print and paper

References

Adult Literacy Support Services (1980) *Understanding labels: problems for poor readers*, Adult Literacy Support Services, London

Aitken-Swan, J. and Easson, E.C. (1959) Reactions of cancer patients on being told their diagnosis. *British Medical Journal, 1*, 779–82

Alfidi, R.J. (1979) Informed consent: a study of patient reaction. *Journal of the American Medical Association, 216*, 1325–9

Alfredsson, L., Bergman, U., Eriksson, R., Gronskog, K., Norell, S.E., Schwartz, E. and Wiholm, B.-E. (1982) Theophyllines three times daily — when are the doses actually taken? — pharmokinetic ideals versus clinical practice. *European Journal of Respiratory Diseases, 63*, 234–8

Alfredsson, L.S. and Norell, S.E. (1981) Spacing between doses on a thrice daily regimen. *British Medical Journal, 282*, 1036

Anderson, J.L., Dodman, S., Kopelman, M. and Fleming, A. (1979) Patient information recall in a rheumatology clinic. *Rheumatology and Rehabilitation, 18*, 18–22

Anderson, K.O. and Masur, F. (1983) Psychological preparation for invasive medical and dental procedures. *Journal of Behavioral Medicine, 6*, 1–40

Andrasik, F. and Murphy, W.D. (1977) Assessing the readability of thirty-nine behavior-modification training manuals. *Journal of Applied Behavior Analysis, 10*, 341–4

Arnhold, R.G. Adebonojo, F.O., Callas, E.R., Carte, E. and Stein, R.C. (1970) Patients and prescriptions; comprehension and compliance with medical instructions in a suburban medical practice. *Clinical Pediatrics, 9*, 648–51

Ausburn, L. (1981) Patient compliance with medication regimes. In J.L. Sheppard (ed.), *Advances in behavioural medicine. Vol. 1.* Cumberland College, Sydney

Avorn, J., Chen, M. and Hartley, R. (1982) Scientific verus commercial sources of influence on the prescribing behavior of physicians. *American Journal of Medicine, 73*, 4–8

Avorn, J. and Sumerai, S.B. (1983) Improving drug therapy through educational outreach. *New England Journal of Medicine, 308*, 1457–63

Azrin, N.H. and Powell, J. (1969) Behavioral engineering: the use of response priming to improve prescribed self-medication. *Journal of Applied Behavior Analysis, 2*, 39–42

Bain, D.J.G. (1977) Patient knowledge and the content of the consultation in general practice. *Medical Education, 11*, 347–50

Baksas, I. and Helgeland, A. (1980) Patient reaction to information and motivation factors in long term treatment with anti-hypertensive drugs. *Acta Medica Scandinavica, 207*, 407–12

Bales, R.F. (1950) *Interaction process analysis: a method for the study of small groups.* Addison-Wesley, Cambridge, Mass.

Barofsky, I. and Connelly, C.E. (1983) Problems in providing effective care for the chronic psychiatric patient. In I. Barofsky and R.D. Budson (eds), *The chronic psychiatric patient in the community.* SP Medical and Scientific Books, New York

Bartlett, E.E., Grayson, M., Barker, R., Levine, D.M., Golden, A. and Libber, S. (1984) The effects of physician communications skills on patient satisfaction, recall and adherence. *Journal of Chronic Diseases, 37,* 755–64

Bauman, J.B., Reiss, M. and Bailey, J.S. (1984) Increasing appointment keeping by reducing the call–appointment interval. *Journal of Applied Behavior Analysis, 17,* 295–301

Becker, M.H. (1976) Socio-behavioral determinants of compliance. In D.L. Sackett and R.B. Haynes (eds), *Compliance with therapeutic regimens.* Johns Hopkins University Press, Baltimore

Becker, M.H. (1979) Understanding patient compliance. In S.J. Cohen (ed.), *New directions in patient compliance.* Lexington Books, Lexington, Mass.

Becker, M.H., Maiman, L.A., Kirscht, J.P., Haefner, D.P., Drachman, R.H. and Taylor, D.W. (1979) Patient perceptions and compliance: recent studies of the Health Belief Model. In R.B. Haynes, D.W. Taylor and D.L. Sackett (eds), *Compliance in health care.* Johns Hopkins University Press, Baltimore

Becker, M.H., Radius, S.M. and Rosenstock, I.M. (1978) Compliance with a medical regimen for asthma: a test of the Health Belief Model. *Public Health Reports, 93,* 268–77

Bendick, M. and Cantu, M.C. (1978) The literacy of welfare clients. *Social Services Review,* March, 56–68

Benjamin-Bauman, J., Reiss, M.L. and Bailey, J.S. (1984) Increasing appointment keeping by reducing the call–appointment interval. *Journal of Applied Behavior Analysis, 17,* 295–301

Bennett, A.E. (ed.) (1976) *Communication between doctors, nurses and patients.* Oxford University Press, Oxford

Bennett, H.L. (1983) Remembering drink orders: the memory skills of cocktail waitresses. *Human Learning, 2,* 157–69

Bergler, J.H., Pennington, A.C., Metcalfe, M. and Freis, E.D. (1980) Informed consent: how much does the patient understand. *Clinical Pharmacology and Therapeutics, 27,* 435–40

Bergman, A.B. and Werner, R.J. (1963) Failure of children to receive penicillin by mouth. *New England Journal of Medicine, 268,* 1334–8

Berry, S.H., Kanouse, D.E., Hayes-Roth, B., Rogers, W.H., Winkler, J.D. and Garfinkle, J.B. (1981) *Informing patients about drugs: analysis of alternative designs for flurazepam leaflets.* Rand Corporation, Santa Monica, Ca.

Bertakis, K.D. (1977) The communication of information from physician to patient: a method for increasing retention and satisfaction. *Journal of Family Practice, 5,* 217–22

Blackburn, G.L., Lynch, M.E. and Wong, S.L. (1986) The very low calorie diet. In K.D. Brownell and J.P. Foreyt (eds), *Handbook of eating disorders.* Basic Books, New York

Boreham, P. and Gibson, D. (1978) The informative process in private medical consultations: a preliminary investigation. *Social Science and Medicine, 12*, 408–16

Boyd, J.R., Covington, T.R., Stanaszek, W.F. and Coussons, R.T. (1974) Drug defaulting. Part 2: analysis of non-compliance patterns. *American Journal of Hospital Pharmacy, 31*, 485–91

Boyle, C.M. (1970) Differences between patients' and doctors' interpretations of common medical terms. *British Medical Journal, 2*, 286–9

Bradshaw, P.W., Ley, P., Kincey, J.A. and Bradshaw, J. (1975) Recall of medical advice: comprehensibility and specifity. *British Journal of Social and Clinical Psychology, 14*, 55–62

Brody, D.S. (1980) An analysis of patients' recall of their therapeutic regimen. *Journal of Chronic Diseases, 33*, 57–63

Brooks, M.S., Rennie, D.L. and Sondag, R.F. (1964) Reaction of mothers to literature on child rearing. *American Journal of Public Health, 54*, 801–11

Brook, R.H. and Williams, K.N. (1976) Effect of medical care review on the use of injections. *Annals of Internal Medicine, 85*, 509–15

Butt, H. (1977) A method for better physician–patient communication, *Annals of Internal Medicine, 86*, 478–80

Byrne, J.S. and Long, B.E.L. (1976) *Doctors talking to patients.* HMSO, London

Cacioppo, J.T. and Petty, R.E. (1979) Effects of message repetition and position on cognitive response, recall, and persuasion. *Journal of Personality and Social Psychology, 37*, 97–109

Cameron, R. and Best, J.A. (1987) Promoting adherence to health behavior change interventions: recent finding from behavioral research. *Patient Education and Counselling, 10*, 139–54

Campbell, R.K. and Grisafe, J.A. (1975) Compliance with the Washington State patient information requirement. *Journal of the American Pharmaceutical Association, 15*, 494–5

Caron, H.S. (1985) Compliance: the case for objective measurement. *Journal of Hypertension, 3, (Suppl. 1)*, 11–17

Caron, H.S. and Roth, H.P. (1968) Patient's cooperation with a medical regimen. *Journal of the American Medical Association, 203*, 422–6

Caron, H.S. and Roth, H.P. (1977) An evaluation of a program for teaching clinic patients the rationale of their peptic ulcer regimen. *Health Education Monographs, 5*, 25–49

Carstairs, V. (1970) *Channels of Communication,* Scottish Home and Health Department, Edinburgh

Cartwright, A. (1964) *Human relations and hospital care.* Routledge and Kegan Paul, London

Cartwright, A. (1967) *Patients and their doctors.* Routledge and Kegan Paul, London

Cartwright, A. (1983) Prescribing and the doctor–patient relationship. In D. Pendleton and J. Hasler (eds), *Doctor–patient communication.* Academic Press, London

Cassileth, B.R., Zupkis, R.V., Sutton-Smith, K. and March, V. (1980) Informed consent — why are its goals improperly realised? *New*

183

England Journal of Medicine, 302, 896–900

Castle, M., Wilfert, C.M., Cate, T.R. and Osterhout, S. (1977) Antibiotic use at the Duke University Center. *Journal of the American Medical Association, 237,* 2819–22

Central Health Services Council (1963) *Communications between doctors, nurses and patients,* Her Majesty's Stationery Office, London

Chaves, A.D. (1960) A simple paper strip urine test for para-aminosalicylic acid. *American Review of Respiratory Diseases, 80,* 585–6

Cheadle, A.J. and Morgan, R. (1975) The chronic patient's comprehension and recollection of his own clinical review. *British Journal of Psychiatry, 126,* 258–62

Cochran, S.D. (1984) Preventing medical non-compliance in the outpatient treatment of bipolar affective disorder. *Journal of Consulting and Clinical Psychology, 52,* 873–8

Cochran, S.D. (1986) Compliance with lithium regimens in the treatment of bipolar affective disorders. *Journal of Compliance in Health Care, 1,* 153–70

Cockburn, J., Reid, A.L. and Sanson-Fisher, R.W. (1987) The process and content of general practice consultations that involve prescription of antibiotic agents. *Medical Journal of Australia, 147,* 321–4

Cohen, D., Berner, U. and Dubach, U.C. (1985) Physician compliance in the mangement of hypertensive patients. *Journal of Hypertension, 3, (Suppl. 1),* 73–6

Cole, R. (1979) The understanding of medical terminology used in printed health education materials. *Health Education Journal, 38,* 111–21

Cooper, J.K., Love, D.W. and Raffoul, P.R. (1982) Intentional prescription non-adherence (non-compliance) by the elderly. *Journal of the American Geriatrics Society, 30,* 329–33

Crichton, E.F., Smith, D.L. and Demanuele, F. (1978) Patients recall of medication information. *Drug Intelligence and Clinical Pharmacy, 12,* 591–9

Crome, P., Akehurst, M. and Keet, J. (1980) Drug compliance in elderly hospital in-patients: trial of a Dosett box. *Practitioner, 224,* 782–5

Crome, P., Curl, B., Boswell, M., Corless, D. and Lewis, R.R. (1982) Assessment of a new calendar pack — the 'C-Pak'. *Age and Ageing, 11,* 275–9

Cuisinier, M.C.J., Van Eijk, J.T.M., Jonkers, R. and Dokter, H.J. (1986) Psychosocial care and education of the cancer patient. *Patient Education and Counselling, 8,* 5–16

Dale, E. and Chall, J.S. (1948a) A formula for predicting readability. *Educational Research Bulletin, 27,* 11–20

Dale, E. and Chall, J.S. (1948b) A formula for predicting readability: Instructions. *Educational Research Bulletin, 27,* 27–54

Davis, M.S. (1966) Variations in patients' compliance with doctors' orders. *Journal of Medical Education, 41,* 1037–48

DeCastro, E.J. (1972) Doctor–patient communications. *Clinical Pediatrics, 11,* 86–7

DeDombal, F.T., Leaper, D.J., Horrocks, J.C., Staniland, J. and McCann, A.P. (1974) Human and computer aided diagnosis of abdominal pain: further report with emphasis on performance of clinicians. *British Medical Journal, 1*, 376–80

Deliere, H.M. and Schneider, L.E. (1980) A study of CPR skill retention among trained EMTs-ambulance. *The EMT Journal, 4*, 57–60

Department of Defense (1975) *Report of the Military Health Care Study.* US Govt. Printing Office, Washington, DC (041-014000037-7)

Department of Health and Human Services (1980) Prescription drug products: Patient package insert requirements. *Federal Register, 45*, 60754-817

Department of Health, Education and Welfare (1978) *Pretesting in Cancer Communications.* DHEW (NIH 78-1493), Washington, DC

Department of Health, Education and Welfare (1979) *Readability Testing in Cancer Communications.* DHEW (NIH 79-1689), Washington, DC

Devine, E.C. and Cook, T.D. (1982) A meta-analysis of the effects of psycho-educational interventions on length of postsurgical hospital stay. *Nursing Research, 32*, 267–74

DeWet, B. and Hollingshead J. (1980) Medicine compliance in paediatric outpatients. *South African Medical Journal, 58*, 846–8

Deyo, R.A. and Inui, T.S. (1980) Dropouts and broken appointments: A literature review and agenda for future research. *Medical Care, 18*, 1146–57

DiMatteo, M.R. and DiNicola, D.D. (1982) *Achieving patient compliance: The psychology of the medical practitioners role.* Pergamon Press, New York

DiMatteo, M.R., Prince, L.M. and Taranta, A. (1978) Patients' perceptions of physician behaviour. *Journal of Community Health, 4*, 280–9

Doak, L.G. and Doak, C.C. (1980) Patient comprehension profiles: recent findings and strategies. *Patient Counselling and Health Education, 2*, 101–6

Dolinsky, D., Gross, S., Deutsch, T., Demestihas, E. and Dolinsky, R. (1983) Application of psychological principles to the design of written patient information. *American Journal of Hospital Pharmacy, 40*, 266–71

Doob, L.W. (1953) Effects of initial serial position and attitude upon recall under conditions of low motivation. *Journal of Abnormal and Social Psychology, 48*, 199–214

Doyle, B.J. and Ware, J.E. (1977) Physician conduct and other factors that affect consumer satisfaction with medical care. *Journal of Medical Education, 52*, 793–801

Dunbar, J.M., Marshall, G.D. and Hovell, M.F. (1979) Behavioral strategies for improving compliance. In R.B. Haynes, D.W. Taylor and D.L. Sackett (eds), *Compliance in health care.* Johns Hopkins University Press, Baltimore

Dwyer, F.M. (1971) Colour as an instructional variable. *Audio-visual Communication Research, 4*, 399–415

185

Dwyer, F.M. (1972) *A guide for improving visualised communication.* State College Pennsylvania: State College Learning Services

Dwyer, F.R. and Hammel, R.A. (1978) An experimental study: Patient package inserts and their effect on hypertensive patients. *Urban Health,* 7, 46–7; 56, 59–60

Eaton, M. and Holloway, R.L. (1980) Patient comprehension of written drug information. *American Journal of Hospital Pharmacy,* 37, 240–3

Edwards, M. and Pathy, M.S.T. (1984) Drug counselling in the elderly and predicting compliance. *Practitioner,* 228, 291–300

Eklund, L.H. and Wessling, A. (1976) Evaluation of package enclosures for drug package. *Lakaridningen,* 73, 2319–20

Ellis, D.A., Hopkin, J.M., Leitch, A.G. and Crofton, J. (1979) 'Doctors orders': controlled trial of supplementary, written information for patients. *British Medical Journal,* 1, 456

Epstein, L.H. and Cluss, P.A. (1982) A behavioral medicine perspective on adherence vs long-term medical regimens. *Journal of Consulting and Clinical Psychology,* 50, 950–71

Eraker, S.A. and Politser, P. (1982) How decisions are reached: physician and patient. *Annals of Internal Medicine,* 97, 262–8

Faden, R.R., Beauchamp, T.L. and King, N.M.P. (1986) *A History and theory of informed consent.* Oxford University Press, Oxford.

Falvo, D., Woehlke, P. and Deichmann, T. (1980) Relation of physician behaviour vs patient compliance. *Patient Counselling and Health Education,* 2, 185–8

Feiffel, H. (1963) Death. In N. Farberow (ed.), *Taboo Topics,* Prentice Hall, Englewood Cliffs.

Feinstein, A.R., Wood, H.F., Epstein, J.A., Taranta, A., Simpson, R. and Tursky, E. (1959) A controlled study of three methods of prophylaxis against streptococcal infection in a population of rheumatic children. *New England Journal of Medicine,* 260, 697–702

Felker, D.B. (ed.) (1980) *Document Design: A Review of the Relevant Research,* American Institute for Research, Washington, DC

Fischbach, R.L., Signelo-Bayog, A., Needle, A. and Delbanco, T.L. (1980) The patient and practitioner as co-authors of the medical record. *Patient Counselling and Health Education,* 2, 1–5

Fischoff, B., Lichtenstein, S., Slovic, P., Derby, S.L. and Keeney, R.L. (1981) *Acceptable Risk.* Cambridge University Press, Cambridge

Fischoff, B., Slovic, P. and Lichtenstein, S. (1981) Lay foibles and expert fables in judgements about risks. In T. O'Riordan and R.K. Turner (eds), *Progress in Resource Management and Environmental Planning.* Wiley, Chichester

Fishbein, M. and Ajzen, I. (1975) *Belief, Attitude, Intention and Behavior.* Addison-Wesley, Reading, Mass.

Fisher, A.W. (1971) Patients' evalution of outpatient medical care. *Journal of Medical Evaluation,* 46, 238–42

Fisher, L.A., Scott Johnson, T., Porter, D., Bleich, H.L. and Slack, W.V. (1977) Collection of a clean voided urine specimen: A comparison among spoken, written, and computer-based instruction.

American Journal of Public Health, 67, 640–4

Fitts, W.T. and Ravdin, I.S. (1953) What Philadelphia physicians tell patients with cancer. *Journal of the American Medical Association, 153,* 901–4

Fleckenstein, L. (1977) Attitudes towards patient package inserts. *Drug Information Journal, 11,* 23–9

Fleckenstein, L., Joubert, P., Lawrence, R., Patsner, B., Mazullo, J.M. and Lasagna, L. (1976) Oral contraceptive patient information: A questionnaire survey of attitudes, knowledge, and preferred information sources. *Journal of the American Medical Association, 235,* 1331–6

Flesch, R. (1948) A new readability yardstick. *Journal of Applied Psychology, 32,* 221–33

Fletcher, C.M. (1973) *Communication in Medicine.* Nuffield Provincial Hospitals Trust, London

Food and Drug Administration (1979) Prescription drug products: patient labelling requirements. *Federal Register, 44,* 40016–41

Fordham, S.D. (1978) Increasing patient compliance in preparing for the barium enema examination. *American Journal of Radiology, 133,* 913–15

Francis, V., Korsch, B.M. and Morris, M.J. (1969) Gaps in doctor–patient communication. *New England Journal of Medicine, 280,* 535–40

Frankel, R.M. (1980) Microanalysis and the medical encounter: an exploratory study. In D. Anderson (ed.), *Analytic Sociology, Special Issue: Microanalysis and medicine.*

French, C., Mellor, M. and Parry, L. (1978) Patients' views of the ophthalmic optician. *Ophthalmic Optician, 28,* 784–6

Friedman, H.S. (1970) Physician management of dying patients: An exploration. *Psychiatry and Medicine, 1,* 295–305

Frimon, P.C., Finney, J.W., Rapoff, M.A. and Christopherson, E.R. (1985) Improving pediatric appointment keeping with reminders and reduced response requirements. *Journal of Applied Behavior Analysis, 18,* 315–21

Gass, D.A. and Curry, L. (1983) Physicians' and nurses' retention of knowledge and skill after training in CPR. *Canadian Medical Association Journal, 128,* 550–1

Gates, S.J. and Colborn, D.K. (1976) Lowering appointment failures in a neighborhood health center. *Medical Care, 14,* 263–7

Gatherer, A., Parfit, J., Porter, E. and Vessey, M. (1979) *Is Health Education Effective?* Health Education Council Monograph Series (No. 2), London

Gauld, V.A. (1981) Written advice: compliance and recall. *Journal of the Royal College of General Practitioners, 31,* 553–6

Geersten, H.R., Gray, R.M. and Ward, J.R. (1973) Patient non-compliance within the context of seeking medical care for arthritis. *Journal of Chronic Diseases, 26,* 689–98

George, C.F., Waters, W.E. and Nicholas, J.A. (1983) Prescription information leaflets: a pilot study in general practice. *British Medical Journal, 287,* 1193–6

Gerle, B., Lunden, G. and Sandblom, P. (1960) The patient with inoperable cancer from the psychiatric and social standpoints. *Cancer, 13*, 1206–11

German, P.S., Klein, L.E., McPhee, S.J. and Smith, C.R. (1982) Knowledge of and compliance with drug regimens in the elderly. *Journal of the American Geriatrics Society, 30*, 568–71

Gilbertsen, V.A. and Wangensteen, O.H. (1962) Should the doctor tell the patient the disease is cancer? *Ca: A Cancer Journal for Clinicians, 12*, 82–6

Glanz, K., Kirscht, J.P. and Rosenstock, I.M. (1981) Linking research and practice in patient educations for hypertension: Patient responses in four educational interventions. *Medical Care, 19*, 141–52

Glasgow, R.E., Schafer, L. and O'Neill, H.K. (1981) Self help books and amount of therapist contact in smoking cessation programs. *Journal of Consulting and Clinical Psychology, 49*, 659–67

Gochman, D.S. and Parcel, G.S. (eds) (1982) Children's health beliefs and health behaviors. *Health Education Quarterly, 9*, 104–270

Golodetz, A., Ruess, T. and Michaus, R.L. (1976) The right to know: giving the patient his medical record. *Archives of Physical Medicine and Rehabilitation, 57*, 78–81

Gordis, L, (1969) The inaccuracy of using interviews to estimate patient reliability in taking medicines at home. *Medical Care, 7*, 49–54

Gordis, L. (1979) Conceptual and methodological problems in measuring compliance. In R.B. Haynes, D.W. Taylor and D.L. Sackett (eds), *Compliance in Health Care*, Johns Hopkins University Press, Baltimore

Gordis, L., Desi, L. and Schmerler, H.R. (1976) Treatment of acute sore throats: A comparison of pediatricians and general practitioners. *Pediatrics, 57*, 422–4

Granstrom, P. and Norell, S. (1983) Visual ability and drug regimen. *Acta Ophthalmologica, 61*, 206–19

Greene, B.F. and Neistat, M.D. (1983) Behavior analysis in consumer affairs: Encouraging dental professionals to provide consumers with shielding from unnecessary x-ray exposure. *Journal of Applied Behavior Analysis, 16*, 13–27

Greenwood, R.D. (1973) Should the patient be informed of innocent heart murmurs? *Clinical Pediatrics, 12*, 468–77

Grimm, R.H., Shimoni, K., Harlan, W.R. and Estes, E.H. (1975) Evaluation of patient-care protocol, use by various providers. *New England Journal of Medicine, 302*, 900–2

Grundner, T.M. (1980) On the readability of surgical consent forms. *New England Journal of Medicine, 302*, 900–2

Gunter, B., Berry, C. and Clifford, B. (1982) Remembering broadcast news. *Human Learning, 1*, 13–29

Hagen, R.L. (1974) Group therapy vs behavior therapy in weight reduction. *Behavior Therapy, 5*, 222–34

Hardie, N.R., Gagnon, J.P. and Eckel, F.M. (1979) Feasibility of symbolic directions on prescription labels. *Drug Intelligence and Clinical Pharmacy, 13*, 588–95

Hartley, J. (1980) *The Psychology of Written Communication*, Kogan Page, London

Hartley, J.R. (1982) The psychology of written communication. In D. Canter and S. Canter (eds), *Perspectives on Professional Psychology*, Wiley, Chichester

Haynes, R.B. (1982) Improving patient compliance: an empirical view. In R.B. Stuart (ed.) *Adherence, compliance and generalisation in behavioral medicine.* Brunner-Mazel, New York

Haynes, R.B., Mattson, M.E. and Engebretson, T.O. (eds) (1980a) *Patient compliance to prescribed anti-hypertensive medication regimens: A report of the national heart, lung and blood institute*, National Institutes of Health (NIH 81-2102), Washington, DC

Haynes, R.B., Mattson, M.E., Chobanian, C.V., Dunbar, J.M., Engbretson, D.O., Garrity, T.F., Leventhal, H., Levine, R.J. and Levy, R.L. (1982) Management of compliance in hypertension: report of the NHLBI working group. *Hypertension, 4,* 415–23

Haynes, R.B., Taylor, D.W. and Sackett, D.L. (eds) (1979) *Compliance in health care.* Johns Hopkins University Press, Baltimore

Haynes, R.B., Taylor, D.W., Sackett, D.L., Gibson, E.S., Bernholz, C.D. and Mukherjee, J. (1980b) Can simple clinical measurements direct non-compliance. *Hypertension, 2,* 757–64

Hecht, A.B. (1974) Improving medication compliance by teaching outpatients. *Nursing Forum, 13,* 112–29

Hermann, F. (1973) The out-patient prescription label as a source of medication errors. *American Journal of Hospital Pharmacy, 30,* 155–9

Hermann, F., Herxheimer, S. and Lionel, N.D.W. (1978) Package inserts for prescribed medicines: What minimum information do patients need? *British Medical Journal, 2,* 1132–5

Hetherington, R.R., Ley, P., Spelman, M.S. and Jones, C.C. (1963) *Research into the psychological effects of physical illness.* Unpublished report, Department of Psychiatry, University of Liverpool

Hildreth, H.M. (1946) A battery of feeling and attitude scales for clinical use. *Journal of Clinical Psychology, 6,* 214–21

Hladik, W.B. and White, S.J. (1976) Evaluation of written reinforcement used in counselling cardio-vascular patients. *American Journal of Hospital Pharmacy, 33,* 155–9

Hoelscher, T.J., Lichstein, K.L. and Rosenthal, T.L. (1986) Home relaxation practice in hypertension treatment: Objective assessment and compliance induction. *Journal of Consulting and Clinical Psychology, 54,* 217–21

Hofling, C.K., Brotzman, E., Dalrymple, S., Graves, N. and Pierce, C.M. (1966) An experimental study in nurse–physician relationships. *Journal of Nervous and Mental Diseases, 143,* 171–80

Holcomb, C.A. (1983) The cloze procedure and readability of patient-oriented drug information. *Journal of Drug Education, 13,* 347–57

Horowitz, I.A. (1969) Effects of volunteering, fear arousal, and number of communications on attitude change. *Journal of Personality and Social Psychology, 11,* 34–7

189

Hospital Affiliates International, Inc. (1978) *Hospital Care in America*, Hospital Affiliates International, Nashville, Tenn.

Houghton, M. (1968) Problems in hospital communication. In G. McLachlan (ed.), *Problems and progress in medical care*, Oxford University Press, Oxford

Hugh-Jones, P., Tanser, A.R. and Whitley, C. (1964) Patients' view of admission to a London Teaching Hospital. *British Medical Journal*, 2, 660–4

Hulka, B.S. (1979) Patient–clinician interaction. In R.B. Haynes, D.W. Taylor and D.L. Sackett (eds), *Compliance in health care*, Johns Hopkins University Press, Baltimore

Hulka, B.S., Cassel, J.C., Kupper, L.L. and Burdette, J.A. (1976) Communication, compliance and concordance between physicians and patients with prescribed medications. *American Journal of Public Health*, 66, 847–53

Hulka, B., Kupper, L., Cassel, J., Efird, R. and Burdette, J. (1975a), Medication use and misuse: physician patient discrepancies. *Journal of Chronic Diseases*, 28, 7–21

Hulka, B.S., Kupper, L.L., Cassel, J.C. and Mayo, F. (1975b) Doctor–patient communication and outcomes among diabetic patients. *Journal of Community Health*, 1, 15–27

Hulka, B.S., Kupper, L.L. Cassel, J.C. and Rabineau, R.A. (1975c) Practice characteristics and quality of primary medical care. *Medical Care*, 13, 808–20

Hulka, B.S., Kupper, L.L., Daly, M.B., Cassel, J.C. and Schoen, F. (1975d) Correlates of satisfaction and dissatisfaction with medical care: A community perspective. *Medical Care*, 13, 648–58

Inui, T.S., Carter, W.B., Kukull, W.A. and Haigh, V.H. (1982) Outcome-based doctor–patient interaction analysis. I. Comparison of techniques. *Medical Care*, 20, 535–50

Inui, T.S., Carter, W.B. and Pecoraro, R.E. (1980) Screening for non-compliance among patients with hypertension. *Medical Care*, 18, 986–93

Inui, T.S., Yourtee, E.L. and Williamson, J.W. (1976) Improved outcomes in hypertension after physician tutorials: A controlled trial. *Annals of Internal Medicine*, 84, 646–51

Jaffe, R. (1981) Informed consent about tardive dyskinesia. *Comprehensive Psychiatry*, 22, 434–7

Janis, I.L. (1967) Effect of fear-arousing communications. In L. Berkowitz (ed.), *Advances in experimental social psychology*, Academic Press, New York

Janis, I.L. and Feshbach, S. (1953) Effect of fear-arousing communications. *Journal of Abnormal and Social Psychology*, 48, 78–92

Janz, N.K. and Becker, M.H. (1984) The Health Belief Model: A decade later. *Health Education Quarterly*, 11, 1–47

Jeffery, R.W. and Gerber, W.M. (1982) Group and correspondence treatments for weight reduction. *Behavior Therapy*, 13, 24–30

Jersild, A. (1929) Primacy, recency, frequency and vividness. *Journal of Experimental Psychology*, 12, 58–70

Johnson, J.C. (1975) Stress reduction through sensation information. In

E.G. Sarason and C.D. Spielberger (eds), *Stress and Anxiety, 2,* John Wiley and Sons, New York

Johnson, J.E., Fuller, S.S., Endress, M.P. and Rice, V.H. (1978) Altering patients' response to surgery: an extension and replication. *Research in Nursing and Health, 1,* 111–21

Johnson, J.E. and Leventhal, H. (1974) Effects of accurate expectations and behavioural instructions on reactions during a noxious medical examination. *Journal of Personality and Social Psychology, 29,* 710–18

Jolly, C., Held, B., Caraway, A.F. and Prystowsky, H. (1971) Research in the delivery of female health care: the recipient's reaction. *American Journal of Obstetrics and Gynecology, 110,* 291–4

Jones, W.H.S. (1967) *Hippocrates,* (Vol. 2, p. 297). Heinemann, London

Jones, W.L., McClellan, P., Shani, Z., Pellegrini, R., Grover, P.L. and Eystrom, P.F. (1982) Cancer patients' preferences for education methods and media. In C. Mettlin and G.P. Murphy (eds), *Issues in cancer screening and communications,* Liss, New York

Jonsen, A.R. (1979) Ethical issues in compliance. In R.B. Haynes, D.W. Taylor and D.L. Sackett (eds), *Compliance in health care,* Johns Hopkins University Press, Baltimore

Joubert, P. and Lasagna, L. (1975) Patient package inserts. I: Nature, notions and needs. *Clinical Pharmacology and Therapeutics, 18,* 507–13

Joyce, C.R.B., Caple, G., Mason, M., Reynolds, E. and Matthews, J.A. (1969) Quantitative study of doctor patient communication. *Quarterly Journal of Medicine, 38,* 183–94

Kahneman, D., Slovic, P. and Tversky, A. (eds), (1982) *Judgement under uncertainty: Heuristics and biases.* Cambridge University Press, Cambridge

Kaim-Caudle, P.R. and Marsh, G.N. (1975) Patient satisfaction survey in general practice. *British Medical Journal, 1,* 262–4

Kalish, R. and Reynolds, D. (1976) *Death and ethnicity: a psychocultural study.* University of Southern California Press, Los Angeles

Kanouse, D.E., Berry, S.H., Hayes-Roth, B., Rogers, W.H. and Winkler, J.D. (1981a) *Informing patients about drugs: Summary Report.* Rand Corporation, Santa Monica, Ca.

Kanouse, D.E., Berry, S.H., Hayes-Roth, B., Rogers, W.H., Winkler, J.D. and Garfinkle, J.B. (1981b) *Informing patients about drugs: Analysis of alternative designs for estrogen leaflets.* Rand Corporation, Santa Monica, Ca.

Kanouse, D.E. and Hayes-Roth, B. (1980) Cognitive considerations in the design of product warnings. In L.A. Morris, M. Mazzis and I. Barofsky (eds), *Banbury Report 6: Product labelling and health risks.* Cold Spring Harbor Laboratories, Cold Spring Harbor, New York

Kelly, W.D. and Friesen, S.R. (1950) Do cancer patients want to be told? *Surgery, 27,* 822–6

Kendrick, R. and Bayne, J.R.D. (1982) Compliance with prescribed medication by elderly patients. *Canadian Medical Association*

Journal, 127, 961–2

Kennedy, B.J. and Lillehaugen, A. (1979) Patient recall of informed consent. *Medical and Pediatric Oncology, 7,* 173–8

Kennel, J.H., Soroker, E., Thomas, P. and Wasman, M. (1969) What parents of patients with rheumatic fever don't know about the disease and its treatment. *Pediatrics, 43,* 160–7

Kiernan, P.J. and Isaacs, J.B. (1981) Use of drugs in the elderly. *Journal of the Royal Society of Medicine, 74,* 196–200

Kincey, J.A., Bradshaw, P.W. and Ley, P. (1975) Patients' satisfaction and reported acceptance of advice in general practice. *Journal of the Royal College of General Practitioners, 25,* 558–66

King, J. (1983) Health beliefs in the consultation. In D. Pendleton and J. Hasler (eds), *Doctor–patient communication.* Academic Press, London

Kirscht, J.P. and Haefner, D.P. (1973) Effects of repeated threatening health communications. *International Journal of Health Education, 10,* 268–77

Klare, G.R. (1963) *The Measurement of Readability,* Iowa State University Press, Iowa

Klare, G.R. (1974) Assessing readability. *Reading Research Quarterly, 10,* 62–102

Klare, G.R. (1976) A second look at the validity of readability formulas. *Journal of Reading Behavior, 8,* 129–52

Klein, L.E., German, P.S., Levine, D.M., Feroli, E.R. and Ardery, J. (1984) Medication problems amongst outpatients. *Archives of Internal Medicine, 144,* 1185–8

Klein, R. (1979) Public opinion and the National Health Service. *British Medical Journal, 1,* 1296–7

Knapp, D.A., Wolf, H.H., Knapp, D.E. and Rudy, T.A. (1969) The pharmacist as drug advisor. *Journal of the American Pharmaceutical Association, 9,* 502–5 and 543

Koltun, A. and Stone, G.C. (1986) Past and current trends in patient non-compliance research: Focus on diseases, regimens-programs, and provider-disciplines. *Journal of Compliance in Health Care, 1,* 21–32

Korsch, B.M., Freeman, B. and Negrete, V. (1971) Practical implications of doctor–patient interactions: Analysis for pediatric practice. *American Journal of Diseases of Children, 121,* 110–14

Korsch, B.M., Gozzi, E.K. and Francis, V. (1968) Gaps in doctor–patient communication. *Pediatrics, 42,* 855–71

Korsch, B.M. and Negrete, V. (1972) Doctor–patient communication. *Scientific American, August,* pp. 66–73

Kunin, C.M., Tupasi, T. and Craig, W. (1973) Use of antibiotics. *Journal of Internal Medicine, 79,* 555–60

Kupst, M.J., Dresser, K., Schulman, J.L. and Paul, M.H. (1975) Evaluation of methods to improve communication in the physician–patient relationship. *American Journal of Orthopsychiatry, 45,* 420–9

Larsen, K. and Smith, C.K. (1981) Assessment of non-verbal communication in the patient–physician interview. *Journal of Family Practice, 12,* 481–8

Law, R., and Chalmers, C. (1976) Medicines and elderly people: a general practice survey. *British Medical Journal, 1,* 565–8

Laws, P. (1974) *A consumer's guide to avoiding unnecessary radiation exposure.* Public Citizen Inc., Washington, DC

Lebow, J.E. (1976) Consumer assessment of the quality of medical care. *Medical Care, 12,* 328–37

Leeb, D., Bowers, D.G. and Lynch, J.B. (1976) Observations in the myth of informed consent. *Plastic and Reconstructive Surgery, 58,* 280–2

Leistyna, J.A. and Macaulay, J.C. (1966) Therapy of streptococcal infections. *American Journal of Diseases in Children, 111,* 22–6

Leventhal, H. (1970) Findings and theory in the study of fear communications. In L. Berkowitz (ed.), *Advances in experimental social psychology,* Academic Press, New York

Leventhal, H., Brown, D., Shacham, S. and Engquist, G. (1979) Effects of preparatory information on cold pressor distress. *Journal of Personality and Social Psychology, 37,* 688–714

Leventhal, H., Meyer, D. and Nerenz, D. (1980) The common sense representation of illness danger. In S. Rachman (ed.), *Contributions to medical psychology vol. 2,* Pergamon Press, Oxford

Levy, R. and Claravell, V. (1977) Differential effects of a phone reminder on appointment keeping for patients with long and short between visit intervals. *Medical Care, 15,* 435–8

Levy, R.L. and Loftus, G.R. (1983) Compliance and memory. In P. Morris (ed.), *Everyday memory,* Academic Press, London

Levy, S.M. (1983) The process of death and dying: behavioral and social factors. In T.G. Burish and L.A. Bradley (eds), *Coping with chronic disease,* Academic Press, New York

Ley, P. (1972a) Complaints by hospital staff and patients: a review of the literature. *Bulletin of the British Psychological Society, 25,* 115–20

Ley, P. (1972b) Primacy, rated importance and the recall of medical information. *Journal of Health and Social Behavior, 13,* 311–17

Ley, P. (1973) Communication in the clinical setting. *British Journal of Orthodontics, 1,* 173–7

Ley, P. (1976) Towards better doctor–patient communications: Contributions from social and experiment psychology. In A.E. Bennett (ed.), *Communication between doctors and patients.* Oxford University Press, Oxford

Ley, P. (1977) Psychological studies of doctor–patient communication. In S. Rachman (ed.), *Contributions to medical psychology, vol. 1,* Pergamon Press, Oxford

Ley, P. (1978) Psychological and behavioural factors in weight loss. In G.A. Bray (ed.), *Recent advances in obesity research vol. 2,* Newman Publishing, London

Ley, P. (1979a) Memory for medical information. *British Journal of Social and Clinical Psychology, 18,* 245–56

Ley, P. (1979b) The psychology of compliance. In D.J. Oborne, M.M. Gruneberg and J.R. Eiser (eds.), *Research in psychology and medicine Vol. 2,* Academic Press, London

193

Ley, P. (1981) Professional non-compliance: a neglected problem. *British Journal of Clinical Psychology, 20*, 151–4

Ley, P. (1982a) Studies of recall in medical settings. *Human Learning, 1*, 223–33

Ley, P. (1982b) Giving information to patients. In J.R. Eiser (ed.), *Social psychology and behavioral medicine*. Wiley, New York

Ley, P. (1982c) Understanding, memory, satisfaction and compliance. *British Journal of Clinical Psychology, 21*, 241–54

Ley, P. (1982d) Simplification, adjunct questions and the recall of ophthalmological and pediatric leaflets. Unpublished manuscript

Ley, P. (1983) Patients' understanding and recall in clinical communication failure. In D. Pendleton and J. Hasler (eds.), *Doctor patient communication*. Academic Press, London

Ley, P. (1985) Effectiveness of some psychological treatments for obesity. In S.W. Tongz and P.J.V. Beumont (eds.), *Eating disorders: Prevalence and treatment*, Williams & Wilkins/Adis, Sydney

Ley, P. (1986a) Cognitive variables and non-compliance. *Journal of Compliance in Health Care, 1*, 171–88

Ley, P. (1986b) Obesity. In H. Koch (ed.), *Community clinical psychology*. Croom Helm, London

Ley, P. (1987a) The effects of readability, letter size and use of capitals on reactions of the elderly to an information leaflet about antibiotic medication. Unpublished manuscript

Ley, P. (1987b) A possible method for interpreting the results of meta-analyses of the comparative effectiveness of different treatments. *Behavior Research and Therapy, 25*, 165–6

Ley, P., Bradshaw, P.W., Eaves, D. and Walker, C.M. (1973) A method for increasing patients' recall of information presented by doctors. *Psychological Medicine, 3*, 217–20

Ley, P., Bradshaw, P.W., Kincey, J.A. and Atherton, S.T. (1976a) Increasing patients' satisfaction with communication. *British Journal of Social and Clinical Psychology, 15*, 403–13

Ley, P., Bradshaw, P.W., Kincey, J.A., Couper-Smartt, H.J. and Wilson, M. (1974) Psychological variables in the control of obesity. In W.L. Burland, P.D. Samuel and J. Yudkin (eds), *Obesity*, Churchill-Livingstone, London

Ley, P., Flaherty, B., Smith, F., Martin, J. and Renner, P. (1985) *A comparative study of the effects of two warning messages about volatile substances*, New South Wales. Drug and Alcohol Authority, Sydney

Ley, P., Goldman, M., Bradshaw, P.W., Kincey, J.A. and Walker C. (1972) The comprehensibility of some x-ray leaflets. *Journal of the Institute of Health Education 10*, 47–53

Ley, P., Jain, V.K. and Skilbeck, C.E. (1975) A method for decreasing patients' medication errors. *Psychological Medicine, 6*, 599–601

Ley, P. and Morris, L.A. (1984) Psychological aspects of written information for patients. In S. Rachman (ed.), *Contributions to medical psychology Vol. 3*, Pergamon Press, Oxford

Ley, P., Pike, L.A., Whitworth, M.A. and Woodward, R. (1979) Effects of source, context of communication and difficulty level on the success of health education communications. *Health Education Journal, 38,* 47–52

Ley, P., Skilbeck. C.E. and Tulips, J.C. (1975) Satisfaction, understanding and compliance in a general practice sample. Unpublished manuscript

Ley, P. and Spelman, M.S. (1965) Communications in an out-patient setting. *British Journal of Social and Clinical Psychology, 4,* 114–16

Ley, P. and Spelman, M.S. (1967) *Communicating with the patient.* Staples Press, London

Ley, P., Swinson, R., Bradshaw, P.W. and Kincey, J A. (1974) Satisfaction with communications amongst surgical patients. Unpublished manuscript

Ley, P., Whitworth, M.A., Skilbeck, C.E., Woodward, R., Pinsent, R.J.F.H., Pike, L.A., Clarkson, M.E. and Clark, P.B. (1976b) Improving doctor–patient communication in general practice. *Journal of the Royal College of General Practitioners, 26,* 720–4

Ley, P., Whitworth, M.A., Woodward, R. and Yorke, R. (1977) Effects of sidedness and arousal on willingness to volunteer for a slimming programme. *Health Education Journal, 36,* 67–9

Liguori, S. (1978) A quantitative assessment of the readability of P.P.I.s. *Drug Intelligence and Clinical Pharmacy, 12,* 712–16

Litton-Hawes, E. (1978) A discourse analysis of topic selection in medical interviews. *Sociolinguistic Newsletter, 9,* 25–6

Lovius, J., Lovius, B.B.J. and Ley, P. (1973) Comprehensibility of the literature given to children at a dental hospital. *Journal of Public Health Dentistry, 33,* 23–6

Lowenthal, D.T., Briggs, W.A., Mutterperl, R., Adelman, B. and Creditor, M.A. (1976) Patient compliance for antihypertensive medication: the usefulness of urine assays. *Current Therapeutic Research, 19,* 405–9

Luscher, T.F., Vetter, H., Siegenthaler, W. and Vetter, W. (1985) Compliance in hypertension: Facts and concepts. *Journal of Hypertension, 3, (Suppl. 1),* 3–9

McDonald, C.J. (1977) Protocol based computer reminders, the quality of care and the non-perfectibility of man. *New England Journal of Medicine, 295,* 1351–5

McDonald, C.J. (1979) The computer's role in detecting and reducing physician errors. In S.J. Cohen (ed.), *New directions in compliance research.* Lexington Books, Lexington, Mass.

McDonald, C.J., Hui, S.I., Smith, D.M., Tierney, W.M., Cohen, S.J. Weinberger, M. and McCabe, G.P. (1984) Reminders to physicians from an introspective computer medical record. *Annals of Internal Medicine, 100,* 130–8

McDonald, C.J., Murray, R., Jeris, D., Bharvaga, B., Seeger, J. and Blevins, L. (1977) A computer-based record and clinical monitoring system for ambulatory care. *American Journal of Public Health, 67,* 240–5

MacDonald, E.T., Macdonald, J.B. and Phoenix, M. (1977) Improving drug compliance after hospital discharge. *British Medical Journal, 2,* 618–21

MacDonald-Ross, M. (1978) Graphics in text. In L. Schulman (ed.), *Review of research in education, Vol. 5*, F.E. Peacock, Itasca, Ill.

McGhie, A. (1961) *The patient's attitude to nursing care.* Livingstone, Edinburgh

McKenney, J.M. and Harrison, W.L. (1976) Drug-related hospital admissions. *American Journal of Hospital Pharmacy, 33*, 792–5

McKercher, P.L. and Rucker, T.D. (1977) Patient knowledge and compliance with medication instructions. *Journal of the American Pharmaceutical Association, 17*, 282–91

McLaughlin, H. (1969) Smog grading: a new readability formula. *Journal of Reading, 22*, 639–46

McNeil, B.J., Pauker, S.G., Sox, H.C. and Tversky, A. (1982) On the elicitation of preferences for alternative therapies. *New England Journal of Medicine, 306*, 1259–62

Martin, D.D. and Mead, K.M. (1982) Reducing medication errors in a geriatric population. *Journal of the American Geriatrics Society, 4*, 258–60

Martin, M. (1986) Ageing and patterns of change in everyday memory and cognition. *Human Learning, 5*, 63–74

Mathews, A. and Ridgeway, V. (1984) Psychological preparation for surgery. In A. Mathews and A. Steptoe (eds), *Health care and human behaviour.* Academic Press, London

Mayou, R., Williamson, B. and Foster, A. (1976) Attitudes and advice after myocardial infarction. *British Medical Journal, 1*, 1577–9

Mazis, M., Morris, L.A. and Gordon, E. (1978) Patient attitudes about two forms of printed oral contraceptive information. *Medical Care, 16*, 1045–54

Mazzuca, S.A. (1982) Does patient education in chronic disease have therapeutic value? *Journal of Chronic Diseases, 35*, 521–9

Mazzullo, J.M., Lasagna, L. and Griner, P.F. (1974) Variations in interpretation of prescription instructions. *Journal of the American Medical Association, 227*, 929–31

Meagher, F., O'Brien, E. and O'Malley, K. (1985) Compliance in elderly hypertensives. *Journal of Hypertension, 3, (Suppl. 1)*, 41–3

Mehrabian, A. (1972) *Non-verbal communication.* Holt, Rinehart & Winston, New York

Meichenbaum, D. and Turk, D.C. (1987) *Facilitating treatment adherence: a practitioner's guidebook.* Plenum Press, New York

Meller, W. and Anderson, A. (1976) The effect of appointment reminders on keeping appointments in a core city pediatric outpatient department. *Minnesota Medicine, 59*, 625–7

Melville, K.A. (1979) The influence of general practitioners attitudes on their presenting habits. In D. Oborne, M.M. Gruneberg and J.R. Eiser (eds), *Research in psychology and medicine*, Academic Press, London

Meyerovitz, B.E., Heinrich, R.L. and Schag, C.C. (1983) A competency based approach to coping with cancer. In T.G. Burish and L.A. Bradley (eds), *Coping with chronic disease*, Academic Press, New York

Midgeley, J.M. and Macrae, A.W. (1971) Audiovisual media in general practice. *Journal of the Royal College of General Practitioners, 21,* 346–51

Miller, C.K. and Chansky, N.M. (1972) Psychologists scoring of WISC protocols. *Psychology in the Schools, 9,* 144–52

Miller, C.K., Chansky, N.M. and Gredler, G.R. (1970) Rater agreement on WISC protocols. *Psychology in the Schools, 7,* 190–3

Miller, P.M. and Sims, K.L. (1981) Evaluation and component analysis of a comprehensive weight control program. *International Journal of Obesity, 5,* 57–65

Millstein, L.G. (1985) Issues in geriatric labelling revisions. In S.R. Moore and T.W. Teal (eds), *Geriatric drug use: clinical and social perspectives,* Pergamon Press, New York

Moll, J.M.H. and Wright, V. (1972) Evaluation of the Arthritis and Rheumatism Council handbook on gout. *Annals of the Rheumatic Diseases, 31,* 405–11

Moll, J.M.H., Wright, V., Jeffrey, M.R., Goode, J.D. and Humberstone, P.M. (1977) The cartoon in doctor patient communication. *Annals of the Rheumatic Diseases, 36,* 225–31

Morisky, D.E., Green, L.W. and Levine, D.M. (1986) Concurrent and predictive validity of a self-reported measure of medication adherence. *Medical Care, 24,* 67–74

Morris, L.A. and Groft, S. (1982) Patient package inserts: a research perspective. In K. Melmon (ed.), *Drug therapeutic concepts for clinicians.* Elsevier, New York

Morris, L.A. and Halperin, J. (1979) Effects of written drug information on patient knowledge and compliance: A literature review. *American Journal of Public Health, 69,* 47–52

Morris, L.A. and Kanouse, D.E. (1980) Consumer reactions to differing amounts of written drug information. *Drug Intelligence and Clinical Pharmacy, 14,* 531–6

Morris, L.A. and Kanouse, D.E. (1981) Consumer reactions to the tone of written drug information. *American Journal of Hospital Pharmacy, 38,* 667–71

Morris, L.A. and Kanouse, D.E. (1982) Informing patients about drug side-effects. *Journal of Behavioral Medicine, 5,* 363–74

Morris, L.A., Mazis, M. and Gordon, E. (1977) A survey of the effects of oral contraceptive information. *Journal of the American Medical Association, 238,* 2504–8

Morris, L.A., Myers, A., Gibbs, P. and Lao, S. (1980) Estrogen PPIs: An FDA survey. *American Pharmacy, NS20,* 22–6

Morris, L.A., Myers, A. and Thilman, D.G. (1980) Application of the readability concept to patient–oriented drug information. *American Journal of Hospital Pharmacy, 37,* 1504–9

Morrow, G. (1980) How readable are surgical consent forms. *Journal of the American Medical Association, 244,* 56–8

Morrow, G., Gootnick, J. and Schmale, A. (1978) A simple technique for increasing cancer patients knowledge of informed consent to treatment. *Cancer, 42,* 793–9

Morse, D.L., Coulter, M.P., Nazarian, L.F. and Napodano, R.J. (1981) Waning effectiveness of mailed reminders on reducing broken appointments. *Pediatrics, 68*, 846–9

Moulding, T. (1962) Proposal for a time-recording pill dispenser as a method for studying and supervising the self-administration of drugs. *American Review of Respiratory Diseases, 85*, 754–7

Moulding, T. (1971) The medication monitor for studying the self-administration of oral contraceptives. *American Journal of Obstetrics and Gynecology, 110*, 1143–4

Moulding, T. (1974) Self-administration of isoniazid and thiacetazone studied by the medication monitor. *Chest, 65*, 234–5

Moulding, T. (1979) The unrealised potential of the medication monitor. *Clinical Pharmacology and Therapeutics, 25*, 131–6

Moulding, T., Knight, S.J. and Colson, J.B. (1967) Vertical pill calendar and medication monitor for improving the self-administration of drugs. *Tubercle, 48*, 32–7

Moulding, T., Onstad, D. and Sbarbaro, J.S. (1970) Supervision of outpatient drug therapy with the medication monitor. *Annals of Internal Medicine, 73.* 559–64

Mullen, P.D., Green, L.W. and Persinger, G.S. (1985) Clinical trials of patient education for chronic conditions: A comparative meta-analysis of intervention types. *Preventive Medicine, 14*, 753–81

Mumford, E., Schlesinger, H.J. and Glass, G.V. (1982) The effects of psychological intervention on recovery from surgery and heart attacks: An analysis of the literature. *American Journal of Public Health, 72*, 141–51

Mushlin, A.I. and Appel, F.A. (1977) Diagnosing patient non-compliance. *Archives of Internal Medicine, 137*, 318–21

Muss, H.B., White, D.R., Michelutte, R., Richards, F.H., Cooper, M.R., Williams, S., Stuart, J.T. and Spurr, C.L. (1979) Written informed consent in patients with breast cancer. *Cancer, 43*, 1549–56

Myers, E.D. and Calvert, E.J. (1973) Effects of prewarning on the occurrence of side-effects and discontinuation of medication in patients on amitripyline. *British Journal of Psychiatry, 122*, 461–4

Myers, E.D. and Calvert, E.J. (1976) Effect of prewarning on the occurrence of side-effects and discontinuance of medication in patients on dothiepen. *Journal of International Medical Research, 4*, 237–40

Myers, E.D. and Calvert, E.J. (1978) Knowledge of side-effects and perseverance with medication. *British Journal of Psychiatry, 132*, 526–7

Nazarian, L.F., Mechaber, R.N., Charney, E. and Coulter, M.P. (1974) Effect of a mailed appointment reminder on appointment keeping. *Pediatrics, 53*, 349–52

Newcomer, D.R. and Anderson, R.W. (1974) Effectiveness of a combined drug self administration and patient teaching program. *Drug Intelligence and Clinical Pharmacy, 8*, 374–81

Norell, S.E. (1979) Improving medication compliance: a randomised clinical trial. *British Medical Journal, 2*, 1031–3

Norell, S.E. (1981a) Accuracy of patient interviews and estimates by clinic staff in determining medication compliance. *Social Science and Medicine, 15E*, 57–61

Norell, S.E. (1981b) Spacing between doses on a thrice-daily regimen. *British Medical Journal, 282*, 1036

Norell, S.E. (1982a) Pilocarpine t.i.d. — how is it taken? *Pharmacy International, 3*, 123–5

Norell, S.E. (1982b) Malignant compliance. *Lancet, 1*, 50

Norell, S.E. (1985) Memory and medication compliance. *Journal of Clinical and Hospital Pharmacy, 10*, 107–9

Norell, S.E., Alfredsson, L., Bergman, U., Eriksson, R.C., Gronskog, K.E., Schwartz, E. and Wiholm, B.-E. (1984) Spacing of medications schedules t.i.d. *American Journal of Hospital Pharmacy, 41*, 1183–5

Norell, S.E. and Granstrom, P. (1980) Self-medication with pilocarpine among outpatients in a glaucoma clinic. *British Journal of Ophthalmology, 64*, 137–41

Norell, S.E., Granstrom, P. and Wassen, R. (1980) A medication monitor and fluorescein technique designed to study medication behaviour. *Acta Ophthalmologia, 58*, 459–67

Novack, D.H., Plummer, R., Smith, R.L., Ochtill, H., Morrow, G.R. and Bennett, J. (1979) Changes in physicians' attitudes toward telling cancer patients. *Journal of the American Medical Association, 241*, 897–900

O'Farrell, T.J. and Keuther, N.J. (1983) Readability of behaviour therapy self-help manuals. *Behavior Therapy, 14*, 449–54

Oken, D. (1961) What to tell cancer patients: a study of medical attitudes. *Journal of the American Medical Association, 175*, 1120–8

Olins, N.J. (1985) Pharmacy interventions. In S.R. Moore and T.N. Teal (eds), *Geriatric drug use: Clinical and social perspectives.* Pergamon Press, New York

Park, L.C. and Lipman, R.S. (1964) A comparison of patient dosage deviation reports with pill counts. *Psychopharmacologia, 6*, 299–302

Parkin, D.M. (1976) Survey of the success of communications between hospital staff and patients. *Public Health, London, 90*, 203–9

Parkin, D.M., Henney, C.R., Quirk, J. and Crooks, J. (1976) Deviations from prescribed treatment after discharge from hospital. *British Medical Journal, 2*, 686–8

Paulson, P.T., Bauch, R., Paulson, M.L. and Zilz, D.A. (1976) Medication data sheets — an aid to patient education. *Drug Intelligence and Clinical Pharmacy, 10*, 448–53

Pendleton, D. and Hasler, J. (1983) *Doctor–patient communication.* Academic Press, London

Pezzot-Pearce, T.D., LeBow, M.D. and Pearce, J.W. (1982) Increasing cost-effectiveness in obesity treatment through use of self-help behavioral manuals and decreased therapist contact. *Journal of Consulting and Clinical Psychology, 50*, 448–9

Phillips, W.R. and Little, T.L. (1980) Continuity of care and poisoning prevention education. *Patient Counselling and Health Education*, 170–3

Poulton, E.C. (1969) How efficient is print? *New Society, No. 349*, 869–71

Poulton, E.C., Warren, T.R. and Bond, J. (1970) Ergonomics in journal design. *Applied Ergonomics, 13,* 207–9

President's Commission for the Study of Ethical Problems in Medicine and Biomedical and Behavioral Research (1982) *Making health care decisions.* US Government Printing Office, Washington, DC

Preston, D.F. and Miller, F.L. (1964) The tuberculosis patient's defection from therapy. *American Journal of Medical Science, 247,* 21–5

Priluck, I.A., Robertson, D.M. and Buettner, H. (1979) What patients recall of the preoperative discussion after retinal detachment surgery. *American Journal of Ophthalmology, 87,* 620–3

Pyrczak, F. and Roth, D.H. (1976) Readability of directions on non-precription drugs. *Journal of the American Pharmaceutical Association, 16,* 242–3

Raphael, W. (1969) *Patients and Their Hospitals,* King Edward's Hospital Fund, London

Raphael, W. and Peers, V. (1972) *Psychiatric patients view their hospitals.* King Edward's Hospital Fund, London

Raven, B.H. and Haley, R.W. (1982) Social influence and compliance of hospital nurses with infection control policies. In J.R. Eiser (ed.), *Social psychology and behavioral medicine.* Wiley, New York

Reading, A.E. (1981) Psychological preparations for surgery: patient recall of information. *Journal of Psychomatic Research, 25,* 57–62

Redlich, F.C. (1949) The patient's language. *Yale Journal of Biology and Medicine, 17,* 427–53

Rehder, T.L., McCoy, L.K., Blackwell, B., Whitehead, W. and Robinson, A. (1980) Improving medication compliance by counselling and special prescription container. *American Journal of Hospital Pharmacy, 37,* 379–86

Reiss, M.L. and Bailey, J.S. (1982) Visiting the dentist: a behavioral community analysis of participation in a dental health screening and referral program. *Journal of Applied Behavior Analysis, 15,* 353–62

Rennick, D. (1960) What should physicians tell cancer patients? *New Medical Materials, 2,* 51–3

Reynolds, M. (1978) No news is bad news: patients' views about communication in hospital. *British Medical Journal, 1,* 1673–6

Reynolds, P.M., Sanson-Fisher, R.W., Poole, A.D., Harker, J. and Byrne, M.J. (1981) Cancer and communication: information-giving in an oncology clinic. *British Medical Journal, 282,* 1449–51

Rice, J.M. and Lutzker, J.R. (1984) Reducing non-compliance to follow-up appointment keeping at a family practice center. *Journal of Applied Behavior Analysis, 17,* 303–11

Richardson, J.L. (1986) Perspectives on compliance with drug regimens among the elderly. *Journal of Compliance in Health Care, 1,* 33–45

Rickels, K. and Briscoe, E. (1970) Assessment of dosage deviation in outpatient drug research. *Journal of Clinical Pharmacology, 10,* 153–60

Riley, C.S. (1966) Patients' understanding of doctors' instructions. *Medical Care, 4,* 34–37

Rimer, B., Keintz, M.K. and Glassman, B. (1985) Cancer patient education: reality and potential. *Preventive Medicine, 4,* 801–18

Roberts, A.W. and Visconti, J.A. (1972) The rational and irrational use of systemic anti-microbial drugs. *American Journal of Hospital Pharmacy, 29,* 1054–60

Robinson, G. and Merav, A. (1976) Informed consent: recall by patients tested post-operatively. *Annals of Thoracic Surgery, 22,* 209–12

Roghmann, K.J., Hengst, A. and Zastowny, T.R. (1979) Satisfaction with medical care: Its measurement and relation to utilisation. *Medical Care, 17,* 461–77

Romankiewicz, J., Gotz, V. and Carlin, H. (1978) Innovations in hospital pharmacy practice. *US Pharmacist,* Nov–Dec. H24–H34

Romm, F.J. and Hulka, B.S. (1979) Care process and patient outcomes in diabetes mellitus. *Medical Care, 17,* 748–57

Rosenberg, S.G. (1971) Patient education leads to better care for heart patients. *HSMHA Health Reports, 86,* 793–802

Rosenthal, R. and Rubin, D.B. (1982) A simple general purpose display of magnitude of experimental effect. *Journal of Educational Psychology, 74,* 166–9

Roter, D.L. (1977) Patient participation in the patient–provider interaction: The effects of question asking on the quality of interaction, satisfaction, and compliance. *Health Education Monographs, 5,* 281–315

Roter, D. (1983) Physician–patient communication. *Maryland State Medical Journal, 32,* 260–5

Roth, H.P. (1979) Problems in conducting a study of the effects on patient compliance of teaching the rationale for antacid therapy. In S.J. Cohen (ed.), *New directions in patient compliance,* Lexington Books, Lexington, Mass.

Roth, H.P. and Caron, H.S. (1978) Accuracy of doctors' estimates and patients' statements on adherence to a drug regimen. *Clinical Pharmacology and Therapeutics, 23,* 361–70

Roth, H.P., Caron, H.S. and Hsi, B.P. (1970) Measuring intake of a presented medication: A bottle count and tracer technique compared. *Clinical Pharmacology and Therapeutics, 11,* 228–37

Roth, H.P., Caron, H.S., Ort, R.S., Berger, D.G., Merrill, R.S., Albee, G.W. and Streeter, G.A. (1962) Patients' beliefs about peptic ulcer and its treatment. *Annals of Internal Medicine, 56,* 72–80

Rowles, B., Keller, S.M. and Gavin, P.W. (1974) The pharmacist as compounder and consultant. *Drug Intelligence and Clinical Pharmacy, 8,* 242–4

Sackett, D.L. (1979) A compliance practicum for the busy practitioner. In R.B. Haynes, D.W. Taylor and D.L. Sackett (eds), *Compliance in health care.* Johns Hopkins University Press, Baltimore

Sackett, D.L. and Haynes, R.B. (eds), (1976) *Compliance with therapeutic regimens.* Johns Hopkins University Press, Baltimore

Sackett, D.L., Haynes, R.B., Gibson, E.S., Hackett, B.C., Taylor, D.W., Roberts, R.S. and Johnson, A.L. (1975) Randomised clinical trial of strategies for improving medication compliance in primary hypertension. *Lancet, I,* 1205–7

Sackett, D.L. and Snow, J.C. (1979) Magnitude of compliance and non-compliance. In R.B. Haynes, D.W. Taylor and D.L. Sackett (eds), *Compliance in health care.* Johns Hopkins University Press, Baltimore

Sanazaro, P.J. (1985) A survey of patient satisfaction, knowledge and compliance. *Western Journal of Medicine, 142,* 703–5

Scheckler, W.E. and Bennett, J.V. (1970) Antibiotic usage in seven community hospitals. *Journal of the American Medical Association, 213,* 264–7

Schwartz, D., Wang, M., Zeitz, L. and Goss, M.E.W. (1962) Medication errors made by elderly, chronically ill patients. *American Journal of Public Health, 52,* 2018–29

Schwartz, W.B. (1979) Decision analysis: a look at the chief complaints. *New England Journal of Medicine, 300,* 556–9

Seaman, J.E., Greene, B.F. and Watson-Perczel, M. (1986) A behavioral system for assessing and training cardiopulmonary resuscitation skills among emergency medical technicians. *Journal of Applied Behavior Analysis, 19,* 125–35

Sheiner, L., Rosenberg, B., Marathe, V. and Peck, C. (1974) Differences in serum digoxin concentrations between outpatients and inpatients: An effect of compliance? *Clinical Pharmacology and Therapeutics, 15,* 239–46

Shepard, D.S. and Moseley, T.A.E. (1976) Mailed versus telephoned appointment reminders to reduce broken appointments in a hospital out-patient department. *Medical Care. 14,* 268–73

Shmarak, K.L. (1971) Reduce your broken appointment rate. *American Journal of Public Health, 61,* 2400–4

Shoham-Salomon, V. and Rosenthal, R. (1987) Paradoxical interventions: A meta-analysis. *Journal of Consulting and Clinical Psychology, 55,* 22–8

Skilbeck, C.E., Tulip, J.G. and Ley, P. (1977) Effects of fear arousal, fear exposure and sidedness on compliance with dietary instruction. *European Journal of Social Psychology, 7,* 221–49

Slovic, P., Fischoff, B. and Lichtenstein, S. (1980) Informing people about risk. In L.A. Morris, M.B. Mazis and I. Barofsky (eds), *Product labelling and health risks: Banbury Report, 6,* Cold Spring Harbor Laboratory, Cold Spring Harbor, New York

Smith, C.K., Polis, E. and Hadac, R.R. (1981) Characteristics of the initial medical interview associated with patient satisfaction and understanding. *Journal of Family Practice, 12,* 283–8

Smith, M.L., Glass, G.V. and Miller, T.I. (1980) *The benefits of psychotherapy.* Johns Hopkins University Press, Baltimore

Smith, N.A., Ley, P., Seale, J.P. and Shaw, J. (1987) Health beliefs, satisfaction, and compliance. *Patient Education and Counselling, 10,* 279–86

Smith, N.A., Seale, J.P., Ley, P., Shaw, J. and Bracs, P.U. (1986) Effects of intervention on medication compliance in children with asthma. *Medical Journal of Australia, 144,* 119–22

Smith, P. and Andrews, J. (1983) Drug compliance not so bad, knowledge not so good — the elderly after discharge. *Age and Ageing, 12,* 336–42

Snowman, J. and Cunningham, D.J. (1975) A comparison of pictorial and written adjunct aids. *Journal of Educational Psychology*, *67*, 307–11

Spelman, M.S. and Ley, P. (1966) Knowledge of lung cancer and smoking habits. *British Journal of Social and Clinical Psychology*, *5*, 207–10

Spelman, M.S., Ley, P. and Jones, C.C. (1966) How do we improve doctor–patient communications in our hospitals. *World Hospitals*, *2*, 126–34

Spriet, A., Beiler, D., Dechorgnat, J. and Simon, P. (1980) Adherence of elderly patients to treatment with pentoxifylline. *Clinical Pharmacology and Therapeutics*, *27*, 1–8

Stanley, B., Guido, J., Stanley, M. and Shortell, D. (1984) The elderly patient and informed consent. *Journal of the American Medical Association*, *252*, 1302–6

Stevens, D.P., Staff, R.N. and Mackay, I.R. (1977) What happens when hospitalised patients see their records. *Annals of Internal Medicine*, *86*, 474–7

Stiles, W.B. (1978) Verbal response modes and dimensions of interpersonal roles: a method of discourse analysis. *Journal of Personality and Social Psychology*, *36*, 693–704

Stiles, W.B., Putnam, S.M., Wolf, M.H. and James, S.A. (1979) Interaction exchange structure and patient satisfaction with medical interviews. *Medical Care*, *17*, 667–79

Stimson, G. (1974) Obeying doctors' orders: A view from the other side. *Social Science and Medicine*, *8*, 97–104

Stokes, M. (1978) The reliability of readability formulae. *Journal of Research in Reading*, *1*, 21–34

Stunkard, A.J. (1979) Behavioral medicine and beyond. The example of obesity. In O.F. Pomerleau and J.P. Brady (eds), *Behavioral Medicine: Theory and Practice*. Williams & Wilkins, Baltimore

Sutton, S.R. (1982) Fear arousing communications: a critical examination of research and theory. In J.R. Eiser (eds), *Social psychology and behavioral medicine*. Wiley, New York

Sutton, S.R. and Eiser, J.R. (1974) The effect of fear-arousing communications on cigarette smoking. An expectancy value approach. *Journal of Behavioral Medicine*, *7*, 13–34

Suveges, L. (1977) Impact of counselling by the pharmacist on patient knowledge and compliance. *Proceedings of the McMaster symposium on compliance with therapeutic regimens*. McMaster University, Hamilton, Ontario

Svarstad, B.L. (1974) *The doctor–patient encounter*. Unpublished Ph.D. Thesis, University of Wisconsin

Tagliacozzo, D.M. and Ima, K. (1970) Knowledge of illness as a predicter of patient behavior. *Journal of Chronic Diseases*, *22*, 765–75

Taub, H.A. and Baker, M.T. (1983) The effect of repeated testing upon comprehension of informed consent materials by elderly volunteers. *Experimental Aging Research*, *9*, 135–8

Taylor, C.B., Agras, W.S., Schneider, J.A. and Allen, R.A. (1983) Adherence to instructions to practice relaxation exercises. *Journal of

Consulting and Clinical Psychology, 51, 952–3

Taylor, W.L. (1953) Cloze procedure: a new tool for measuring readability. *Journalism Quarterly, 30,* 415–33

Thomas, J.E. (1979) The relationship between knowledge about food and nutrition and food choice. In M. Turner (ed.), *Nutrition and Lifestyles.* Applied Science Publishers, London

Thrush, R.S. and Lanese, R.R. (1962) The use of printed material in diabetes education. *Diabetes, 11,* 132–7

Tierney, W.M., Hui, S.L. and McDonald, C.J. (1986) Delayed feedback of physician performance versus immediate reminders to perform preventive care: effects on physician compliance. *Medical Care, 24,* 659–66

Tinker, M.A. (1963) *Legibility of Print,* Iowa State University Press, Ames, Iowa

Tinker, M.A. (1966) Experimental studies on the legibility of print. *Reading Research Quarterly, 1,* 67–118

Tring, F.C. and Hayes-Allen, M.C. (1973) Understanding and misunderstanding of some medical terms. *British Journal of Medical Education, 7,* 53–9

Tuckett, D.A., Boulton, M. and Olson, C. (1985) A new approach to the measurement of patients' understanding of what they are told in medical consultations. *Journal of Health and Social Behavior, 26,* 27–38

Tuckett, D.A., Boulton, M., Olson, C. and Williams, A. (1986) *Meetings between experts: an approach to sharing ideas in medical consultations.* Tavistock Publications, London

Tversky, A. and Kahneman, D. (1981) The framing of decisions and the rationality of choice. *Science, 211,* 453–8

Udkow, G.P., Lasagna, L., Weintraub, M. and Tamoshunas, Z. (1979) The safety and efficacy of the patient package insert: A questionnaire study. *Journal of the American Medical Association, 242,* 536–9

United Manchester Hospitals (1970) *Patient satisfaction survey 1968–69.* Patients' Services Committee, United Manchester Hospitals.

US Department of Commerce (1980) *Educational Attainment in the United States: March 1979 and March 1978.* Current Population Reports, Series P-20 No. 356. Washington, DC

Visser, A.P. (1980) Effects of an information booklet on well-being of hospital patients. *Patient Counselling and Health Education, 2,* 51–64

Wagenaar, W.A. (1978) Recalling messages broadcast to the general public. In M.M. Gruneberg, P.E. Morris and R.N. Sykes (eds), *Practical aspects of memory.* Academic Press, London

Wagenaar, W.A., Schreuder, R. and Wijlhuizen, G.J. (1987) Readability of instructional text written for the general public. *Applied Cognitive Psychology, 1,* 155–68

Wallace, L.M. (1986) Communication variables in the design of presurgical preparatory information. *British Journal of Clinical Psychology, 25,* 111–18

Wandless, I. and Davie, J.W. (1977) Can drug compliance in the elderly be improved? *British Medical Journal, 1,* 359–61

Ware, J.W. and Snyder, M.K. (1975) Dimensions of patient attitudes regarding doctors and medical care services. *Medical Care, 13,* 669–82

Wartman, S.A., Morlock, L.L., Malitz, F.E. and Palm, E.A. (1983) Patients' understanding and satisfaction as predictors of compliances. *Medical Care, 21,* 886–91

Watkins, J.D., Williams, T.F., Martin, D.A., Hogan, M.D. and Anderson, E. (1967) A study of diabetic patients at home. *American Journal of Public Health, 57,* 452–9

Watkins, R.L. and Norwood, G.J. (1978) Pharmacist drug consultation behaviour. *Social Science and Medicine, 12,* 235–9

Weaver, F.J., Ramirez, A.G., Dorfman, S.B. and Raizner, A.E. (1979) Trainees' retention of CPR: How quickly they forget. *Journal of the American Medical Association, 241,* 901–3

Webb, B. (1976) The retail pharmacist and drug treatment. *Journal of the Royal College of General Practitioners, 26, Suppl. 1,* 81–8

Weibert, R. (1977) Potential distribution problems. *Drug Information Journal, 11,* 455–95

Wertheimer, A.I., Shefter, E. and Cooper, R.M. (1973) More on the pharmacist as a drug consultant. *Drug Intelligence and Clinical Pharmacy, 7,* 58–61

Wilkins, A.J. and Baddeley, A.D. (1978) Remembering to recall in everyday life: An approach to absent-mindedness. In M.M. Gruneberg, P.E. Morris, and R.N. Sykes (eds), *Practical aspects of memory.* Academic Press, London

Willows, D.M. (1978) A picture is not always worth a thousand words. *Journal of Educational Psychology, 70,* 255–62

Wing, R. and Jeffery, R.N. (1979) Out-patient treatment of obesity: a comparison of methodology and clinical results. *International Journal of Obesity, 3,* 261–79

Winkler, J.D., Kanouse, D.E., Berry, S.H., Hayes-Roth, N., Rogers, W.H. and Garfinkle, J.B. (1981) *Informing patients about drugs: Analysis of alternative designs for erythromycin leaflet.* Rand Corporation, Santa Monica, CA

Wolf, M.H., Putnam, S.M., James, S.A. and Stiles, W.B. (1978) The Medical Interview Satisfaction Scale: Development of a scale to measure patient perceptions of physician behavior. *Journal of Behavioral Medicine, 1,* 391–401

Wright, G. (1984) *Behavioural Decision Theory.* Penguin Books, Harmondsworth

Wright, P. (1977) Presenting technical information: a survey of research findings. *Instructional Science, 6,* 93–134

Wright, P. (1978) Feeding the information eaters: suggestions for integrating pure and applied research on language comprehension. *Instructional Science, 7,* 249–312

Wright, P. (1983) Writing and reading technical information. In J. Nicholson and B. Foss (eds), *Psychology Survey: No. 4.* British Psychological Society, Leicester

Yee, R.D., Hahn, P.M. and Christensen, R.E. (1974) Medication monitor for ophthalmology. *American Journal of Ophthalmology*, *77*, 774–8

Young, L. and Humphrey, M. (1985) Cognitive methods of preparing women for hysterectomy: Does a booklet help? *British Journal of Clinical Psychology*, *24*, 303–4

Index